The hands-on guide
for house officers

D1078150

The hands-on guide for house officers

ANNA DONALD
BA, BM, BCh (Oxon), MPP (Harvard), BA (Sydney)

MICHAEL STEIN
MB ChB, BSc (Hons) (UCT), DPhil (Oxon)

With VIVEK MUTHU
BM, BCh (Oxon), MA (Cantab)

SECOND EDITION

Blackwell
Science

© 1996, 2002 by Blackwell Science Ltd
a Blackwell Publishing Company
Editorial Offices:
Osney Mead, Oxford OX2 0EL, UK
   Tel: +44 (0)1865 206206
Blackwell Science, Inc., 350 Main Street, Malden, MA 02148-5018, USA
   Tel: +1 781 388 8250
Blackwell Science Asia Pty, 54 University Street, Carlton, Victoria 3053, Australia
   Tel: +61 (0)3 9347 0300
Blackwell Wissenschafts Verlag, Kurfürstendamm 57, 10707 Berlin, Germany
   Tel: +49 (0)30 32 79 060

The right of the Authors to be identified as the Authors of this Work has been assert-
ed in accordance with the Copyright, Designs and Patents Act 1988.

All rights reserved. No part of this publication may be reproduced, stored in a re-
trieval system, or transmitted, in any form or by any means, electronic, mechanical,
photocopying, recording or otherwise, except as permitted by the UK Copyright,
Designs and Patents Act 1988, without the prior permission of the publisher.

First published 1996
Second edition 2002

Library of Congress Cataloging-in-Publication Data

Donald, Anna.
    The hands-on guide for house officers / Anna Donald, Michael Stein, with
Vivek Muthu—2nd ed.
        P.   cm.
    Includes bibliographical references and index.
    ISBN 0-632-05331-3 (pbk.)
        1. Residents (Medicine)—Handbooks, manuals, etc.
        2. Medicine—Handbooks, manuals, etc.
        I. Stein, Michael, DPhil.   II. Muthu, Vivek.   III. Title.

RA972 .D66 2002
616—dc21

                                                    2001056461

ISBN 0-632-05331-3

A catalogue record for this title is available from the British Library

Set in 8/9.5 Erhardt by SNP Best-set Typesetter Ltd., Hong Kong
Printed and bound in Great Britain by MPG Books Ltd, Bodmin, Cornwall

For further information on Blackwell Science, visit our website:
www.blackwell-science.com

Contents

Introduction, xi

How to use this book, xii

Acknowledgements, xiii

Abbreviations, xiv

1 Starting up, 1
Panic?, 1
    people to help you, 1
    three basic tips, 2
Other useful start-up
        information, 2
    bibliography, 2
    dress, 3
    equipment, 3
    geography, 4
    ward rounds, 4
    discharging patients, 6
    work environment, 6

**2 Getting organized (four
    lists and a folder), 8**
Personal folder, 8
Keeping track of patients (List 1),
    8
List of things to do (List 2), 10
Phone numbers (List 3), 10
Firm timetable (List 4), 10

3 Paperwork, 11
Patient notes, 11
Accident forms, 11
Blood forms and requesting
        bloods, 12
Consent, 13
Death and cremation certificates,
    13

Discharge summaries
        (TTO/TTA), 13
Drug charts, 14
Drug prescriptions, 14
Handovers, 14
Hand backs, 14
Referral letters, 14
Self-discharge, 15
Sick notes, 15

**4 Accident and
    emergency, 16**
General, 16
Admitting and allocating
        patients, 16
Keeping track of patients, 17
Medicine, 17
Overdose, 17
    treating the patient, 18
Surgery, 21

**5 Becoming a better
    doctor, 23**
Computers, 23
    hardware, 23
    software, 24
    access to on-line databases, 25
A bit about the Internet, 25
Keeping up with the literature, 26
Evidence based medicine, 27
Professionalism, 28
Communication, 28
    consultants and senior
        registrars, 29
    GPs, 30
    nurses, 30
    patients, 32
    patients' families, 32

Confidentiality, 33
   exceptions to keeping
     confidentiality, 34
Consent, 34

**6 Cardiac arrests and crash
calls, 35**
'Do not resuscitate' orders, 37

7 Common calls, 38
How to use this section, 38
Considerations for all ward
   calls, 38
Abdominal pain, 39
Anaemia, 40
Arrhythmia, 42
   initial management for all
     arrhythmias, 42
   managing specific
     arrhythmias, 42
Calcium, 45
   hypercalcaemia, 45
   hypocalcaemia, 46
Chest pain, 47
Confusion, 48
Constipation, 50
Diarrhoea, 51
Electrocardiograms, 52
   important ECG abnormalities
     to recognize, 55
Eye complaints, 56
   the acute red eye, 56
   sudden loss of vision, 57
   floaters, 57
Falls, 57
Fever, 58
   the immunocompromised
     patient with fever, 60
Fits, 60
Intravenous fluids, 62
   how to prescribe IV fluids, 62
Upper gastrointestinal bleeds, 63
   high risk and hypovolaemic
     patients, 64

   low risk patients, 65
Lower gastrointestinal bleeds, 65
Glucose, 65
Gynaecological calls, 66
   vaginal bleeding, 67
   dysmenorrhoea, 67
Haematuria, 67
Headaches, 68
Hypertension, 70
Hypotension, 71
Insomnia, 72
   management with
     benzodiazepines, 73
Itching, 74
Immunocompromised (see Fever)
The moribund patient, 74
Nausea and vomiting, 76
Oliguria/anuria (see Urine, low
   output)
Oxygen therapy, 77
   methods of oxygen delivery, 77
   pulse oximetry, 78
Phlebitis, 78
   management, 78
Potassium, 79
   hyperkalaemia, 79
   hypokalaemia, 79
Rashes and skin lesions, 81
   disease categories, 81
Red eye (see Eye complaints)
Shortness of breath, 82
The sick patient, 84
Sodium, 84
   hyponatraemia, 84
Transfusions, 85
   blood, 85
   platelet, 86
   reactions, 87
Urine, low output, 87
Basic emergency routine, 88

8 Death and dying, 90
Terminal care, 90
Communication, 90

breaking bad news, 90
ongoing communication with
    dying patients, 91
Pain control, 93
Symptom control, 93
Prescribing for the dying, 93
Support for the dying and for
    you, 93
Death, 94
What to do when a patient dies,
    94
Telling relatives about the
    patient's death, 95
Post mortems, 95
Death certificates, 95
    writing the death certificate, 95
Referring to the coroner, 96
Cremation forms and fees, 97
    to check for pacemakers, 97
Further reading, 98

9 Drugs, 99
General, 99
Prescribing drugs, 99
    drug charts, 99
    writing prescriptions, 100
    controlled drugs, 100
    verbals, 101
Giving drugs, 101
    drug infusions, 102
    intravenous drugs, 103
Specific drug topics, 105
    antibiotics, 105
    anticoagulation, 105
    fluid question, 106
    digoxin, 106
    night sedation, 107
    therapeutic drug levels, 107
    steroids, 107
Miscellaneous tips, 107

10 Handle with care, 109
Alcoholism, 109
    alcohol withdrawal, 109

Children, 110
Depression, 110
Elderly patients, 111
Haemophiliacs, 111
    taking blood, 112
    for theatre, 112
HIV/AIDS, 112
    taking blood, 112
    HIV testing, 113
Jehovah's Witnesses/Christian
    Scientists, 113
Pregnant women, 114
Sickle cell anaemia, 114
The steroid patient, 115
    side effects of steroids, 115
    managing ill patients on
        steroids, 115
    treating common side effects,
        116
    withdrawing steroid therapy,
        116

**11 Approach to the medical
    patient, 117**
History and examination, 118
Clinical stalemate, 118
Preparing patients for medical
        procedures, 121
    cardiac catheterization, 121
    elective DC cardioversion, 122
    upper gastrointestinal
        endoscopy, 123
    colonoscopy, 124
    flexible sigmoidoscopy, 124
    liver biopsy, 125
    pericardial aspiration, 125
    renal biopsy, 126
Specialist referrals, 127
    cardiology, 127
    endocrinology, 128
    gastroenterology, 129
    haematology, 130
    neurology, 130
    renal medicine, 131

respiratory medicine, 131
rheumatology, 132

12 Pain, 133

Pain control, 133
general, 133
Specific analgesics, 133
inhaled drugs, 133
oral drugs, 133
IM/IV opiates, 136
other, 138
Pain control by severity and
underlying condition, 138

13 Practical procedures, 140

general hints, 140
Arterial blood gases, 140
interpreting arterial blood
gases, 142
respiratory disease and arterial
blood gases interpretation,
144
Ascitic tap (see Peritoneal tap)
Bladder catheterization, 145
men, 145
women, 146
Blood cultures, 146
Blood letting, 147
Cannulation, 148
Central lines, 151
insertion of central lines, 151
problems with temporary and
tunnelled central lines, 154
using central lines, 155
measuring the CVP, 155
Chest drains, 157
managing a chest drain, 157
how to remove a drain, 158
DC cardioversion, 158
Electrocardiogram, 159
reading ECGs, 161
Exercise stress test, 161
relative contraindications, 161
the procedure, 161

Glucose tolerance test, 161
Injections, 162
subcutaneous, 162
intramuscular, 162
Intercostal block, 162
Joint aspiration/injection, 163
aspiration, 164
injecting joints, 164
Local anaesthesia, 165
Lumbar puncture, 166
Mantoux test, 168
Nasogastric tubes, 169
Peritoneal tap, 169
Pleural aspiration, 171
Pulsus paradoxus, 173
Respiratory function tests, 173
spirometry, 173
peak expiratory flow rate, 175
Sutures, 177

14 Radiology, 178

Requesting investigations, 178
Minimizing radiation, 178
Common concerns about X-rays,
178
Pregnancy, 180
Plain films, 180
chest X-rays before surgery,
180
skull X-rays, 180
abdominal films, 180
Contrast studies, 181
intravenous urography, 181
barium swallow, 182
barium meal, 182
small bowel enema, 182
barium enema, 182
Ultrasound, 182
Computerized tomography, 183
general, 183
CT head, 183
Arteriography, 183
Magnetic resonance imaging, 184
Radioisotope scanning, 184

15 Surgery, 185
Routine clerking, 185
Peri-operative prescribing, 186
Consent, 189
expected side effects after
surgery, 191
Anaesthetics, 191
Drawing up theatre lists, 192
Marking patients for surgery,
192
Post operative care, 192
Complicated patients, 193
jaundice, 193
diabetes, 193
steroid–dependent patients,
195
thyroid surgery, 195
Day surgery, 196
Oro-facio-maxillary surgery, 196
Surgical protocol clerking sheet,
197

16 Self care, 198
Accommodation, 198
Alternative careers, 198
Bleep, 199
British Medical Association
(BMA), 199
Car and insurance, 199
Clothes, 199
Contacting medical colleagues,
200
Contract and conditions of
service, 200
what you need to know about
your contract, 200
Doctors' mess, 204
making money for the mess,
204
Drug representatives, 204
Insurance (room contents), 204
Jobs, 205
curriculum vitae, 205
the interview, 206

consultant career prospects,
206
locums, 206
Meals, 207
Medical defence, 207
Money, 208
income protection, 208
payslip deductions, 208
pensions, 209
tax, 209
telephone and on-line banking,
211
Needlestick injuries, 211
if the patient is known to be
HIV-positive, 211
if the patient is known to be
hepatitis-positive, 212
Not coping, 212
Part-time work, 213
Representation of junior doctors,
213
Sleep, 213

**Appendix A Useful tests,
numbers and other
information, 215**
Addresses, 215
poisons information, 215
Barthel score, 215
Glasgow Coma Scale, 216
Mental Health Act, 216
Mini–mental test score, 217
Notifiable diseases, 217
Results, 218
haematology, 218
how to interpret, 218
Useful biochemical formulae, 219
Fitness to drive, 220

**Appendix B Diagrams for
explaining procedures to
patients, 223**
A1 The thorax, 223
A2 Coronary arteries, 224

A3 Upper gastrointestinal tract, 225
A4 Large intestine, 226
A5 Digestive organs, 227
A6 Female pelvis, 228
A7 Male pelvis, 229

A8 Urinary system, 230
Tunnelled central lines (see Fig. 13.4)

Index, 231

Introduction

Your House Officer year is guaranteed to be one of the big experiences of your life. Free at last from rote learning and endless exams, your house job is intensely practical. The trouble is that the theoretical training in medical school does not usually prepare you for the physical and emotional rigours of hundreds of tasks being thrust upon you around the clock. Similarly, medical textbooks rarely deal with the practical know-how which makes all the difference between clumsy and elegant doctoring.

This book is based on the collective experience of junior doctors who remember only too well the highs and lows of their house job year. It contains information not readily available in standard texts, that will help you to feel competent and confident despite sleepless nights and low blood sugars. It assumes minimal practical know-how. Subjects are listed in alphabetical order within each chapter. A detailed index is also provided for rapid reference.

Whatever you do, keep your head up and keep smiling. Hospitals are funny places. Lots of people love their house job; we hope you are one of them. Take care and good luck!

A.K.D.
M.L.S.
V.S.M.

How to use this book

This book is designed as a user-friendly manual. We would recommend skimming through it when you first buy it, and then referring to relevant sections for particular problems that you come across.

This book provides standard algorithms for diagnosis and management of clinical problems that worked for us and our colleagues, in different settings throughout Britain. Please don't follow our instructions slavishly. We realize that every firm has its own way of doing things and that there may be more appropriate algorithms for specialist wards or unusual situations. Like a recipe book, feel free to scrawl in the margins to make it more usable for you. We have included some blank pages at the back for extra notes. We want to emphasize that this book is not the *Oxford Textbook of Medicine*, so please don't expect to find the 337 causes of tropical swollen legs here!

To keep the book compact and maximally relevant to what you need, we have not attempted to replicate the *BNF*. While we do suggest drugs where relevant, we realized from our own experience that the safest and most efficient way to prescribe drugs is to use the *BNF* in conjuction with your hospital's drug formulary.

Finally, if you discover a better way of doing something, please let us know. A card is included in the book for future suggestions. If we can use your suggestion, you will be acknowledged in the next edition of the book.

Acknowledgements

This book is dedicated to Uncle Ivan Harris; to Bruce, Janet and Tom Donald; and to Marissa, Amit, Sundar and Usha Muthu, for the support and love that made writing this book possible.

There are many people we wish to thank: Ian Crossley for his support and repeated reading of draft manuscripts; Ruariridh Milne for his brilliant ideas, and Solly Benatar, Muir Gray, Tony Hope, Lionel Opie, Antony Rosen, David Sackett and Basil Shepstone for their inspiration in practising medicine. We especially want to thank doctors and nurses at the John Radcliffe Hospital and Glasgow Royal Infirmary for their teaching, and humane and rigorous approach to clinical practice.

We would like to thank Deborah Castle, Matt Collins, Helen Dignum, Andy Eynon, Nicholas Fleming, Judy Mead, Joe Rosenthal, and Wim de Villiers for editing, ideas and contributions from their experience in NHS hospitals and health authorities. We don't know what we would have done without Andy's attention to detail and green ink! Helen Dignum wrote most of the chapter on Self care, read and re-read draft manuscripts and contributed her own hints and corrections to most chapters. Thanks also to Chris Glynn for his contribution to the chapter on Pain control and for his enthusiasm, and to Derek Crook for his generosity and encouragement. Many thanks to Satish Keshav, a true gentleman, scholar and friend, who made invaluable suggestions and wrote the section Clinical Stalemate.

Special thanks to Lisa Stein, for listening without criticizing. To Hyme, Jenny and Nicholas Rabinowitz, for their love and friendship. To Oliver and Rosemary Russell for years of love, care and encouragement, with this book and everything else.

We would also like to thank our dear friends who made suggestions, encouraged, fed and watered us throughout the course of this book: Elleke Boehmer, Wim and Katherine de Villiers, Elizabeth Jardine, Steve Matthews, Sarah Nuttall, Joel, Ai-Zhen and Sara Tatelman.

Finally, to Michael Anderson for his generosity and love, not to mention the chess, tips on grammar and daily care that kept the wheels turning in the last stages of the manuscript.

Fifty per cent of the authors' royalties for this book are donated to the University of Cape Town Medical School.

Abbreviations

We include a long list of abbreviations to aid reading medical notes and for reference throughout this book.

μg	micrograms
−ve	negative
+ve	positive
A&E	Accident and Emergency
ABC	Airway, Breathing, Circulation
ABG	arterial blood gases
ac	*ante cibum* (before food)
ACE	angiotensin-converting enzyme
ACTH	adrenocorticotrophic hormone
ADH	antidiuretic hormone
AF	atrial fibrillation
AFB	acid-fast bacillus
AIDS	acquired immunodeficiency syndrome
ALP (alk phos)	alkaline phosphatase
ALT	alanine aminotransferase
ANA	antinuclear antigen
ANCA	antineutrophil cytoplasmic antigen
ANF	antinuclear factor
APTT	activated partial thromboplastin time
ARC	AIDS-related complex
ARDS	adult respiratory distress syndrome
ARF	acute renal failure
ASAP	as soon as possible
ASD	atrial septal defect
ASOT	antistreptolysin O titre
AST	aspartate transaminase
ATN	acute tubular necrosis
AV	atrioventricular
AVCs	additional voluntary contributions
AXR	abdominal X-ray (plain)
Ba	barium
BBB	bundle branch block
bd	*bis die* (twice per day)
bHCG	beta–human chorionic gonadotrophin
BMA	British Medical Association
BMJ	*British Medical Journal*
BNF	*British National Formulary*
BP	blood pressure
bpm	beats/minute
C&E	creatinine and electrolytes
Ca	carcinoma
Ca	calcium
CABG	coronary artery bypass graft
CBD	common bile duct
CCF	congestive cardiac failure
CCU	coronary care unit
CEA	carcino–embryonic antigen
CFC	complement fixation test
CI	contraindications
CK	creatinine kinase
CK-MB	creatine kinase cardiac isoenzyme
CLL	chronic lymphocytic leukaemia
CML	chronic myeloid leukaemia
CMV	cytomegalovirus
CNS	central nervous system

COAD	chronic obstructive airways disease	FBC	full blood count
CPR	cardiopulmonary resuscitation	FDP	fibrin degradation product
		FEV_1	forced expiratory volume in first second
CRF	chronic renal failure	FFP	fresh frozen plasma
CRP	C-reactive protein	FOB	faecal occult blood
CSF	cerebrospinal fluid	FSH	follicle stimulating hormone
CT	computerized tomography		
CV	curriculum vitae	FVC	forced vital capacity
CVA	cerebrovascular accident	Fx	family
CVP	central venous pressure	g	gram(s)
CVS	cardiovascular system	G&S	group and save
CXR	chest X-ray	G6PD	glucose-6-phosphate dehydrogenase
D&V	diarrhoea and vomiting		
DDAVP	desmopressin	GBM	glomerular basement membrane
DIC	disseminated intravascular coagulation		
		GCS	Glasgow Coma Scale
DIP	distal interphalangeal	GFR	glomerular filtration rate
DKA	diabetic ketoacidosis	GGT	gamma-glutamyl transferase
dl	decilitre(s)		
DM	diabetes mellitus	GH	growth hormone
DNR	do not resuscitate	GI (GIT)	gastrointestinal
DOA	date of admission	GKI	glucose, potassium and insulin
DOB	date of birth		
DOD	date of death	GMC	General Medical Council
DoH	Department of Health	GN	glomerulonephritis
DVLC	Driver and Vehicle Licensing Centre	GP	general practitioner
		GT	glutamyl transferase
DVT	deep venous thrombosis	GTN	glyceryl trinitrate
DXT	radiotherapy	GTT	glucose tolerance test
EBV	Epstein–Barr virus	GU	genito-urinary
ECG	electrocardiogram	HB	heart block
ECHO	echocardiography	Hb	haemoglobin
EDTA	ethylene diamine tetra-acetic acid	HBsAg	hepatitis B surface antigen
		Hct	haematocrit
EEG	electroencephalogram	HDL	high density lipoprotein
ELISA	enzyme-linked immunosorbent assay	HDU	high dependency unit
		Hep	hepatitis
EM	electron microscope	HiB	*Haemophilus influenzae* B vaccine
ENT	ear, nose and throat		
ERCP	endoscopic retrograde cholangiopancreatography	HIV	human immunodeficiency virus
ESR	erythrocyte sedimentation rate	HLA	human leukocyte antigen

HO	House Officer	LBBB	left bundle branch block
HOCM	hypertrophic obstructive cardiomyopathy	LDH	lactate dehydrogenase
		LDL	low density lipoprotein
HPC	history of presenting complaint	LFT	liver function test
		LH	luteinizing hormone
HS	heart sounds	LIF	left iliac fossa
HT	hypertension	LMN	lower motor neurone
IBD	inflammatory bowel disease	LMP	last menstrual period
		LOC	loss of consciousness
IBS	irritable bowel syndrome	LP	lumbar puncture
ICP	intracranial pressure	LUQ	left upper quadrant
ID	identification	LV	left ventricle
IDDM	insulin-dependent diabetes mellitus	LVF	left ventricular failure
		LVH	left ventricular hypertrophy
Ig	immunoglobulin		
IHD	ischaemic heart disease	*mane*	in the morning
IM	intramuscular	MC&S	microscopy, culture and sensitivity
INR	international normalised ratio (prothrombin ratio)		
		MCV	mean cell volume
IPPV	intermittent positive pressure ventilation	MDU	Medical Defence Union
		Mg	magnesium
ISDN	isosorbide di-nitrate	mg	milligrams
ITP	idiopathic thrombocytopenic purpura	MI	myocardial infarction
		ml	millilitres
		mmHg	millimetres of mercury
ITU	intensive therapy unit	MND	motorneurone disease
iu (IU)	international unit	MPS	Medical Protection Society
IUCD	intrauterine contraceptive device		
		MRI	magnetic resonance imaging
IV	intravenous		
IVC	inferior vena cava	MRSA	methicillin resistant *Staphylococcus aureus*
IVI	intravenous infusion		
IVU	intravenous urography	MS	multiple sclerosis
JAMA	*Journal of the American Medical Association*	MSK	musculoskeletal
		MST	morphine sulphate tablets
JVP	jugular venous pressure		
K^+	potassium	MSU	midstream urine
KCCT	kaolin-cephalin clotting time	N&V	nausea and vomiting
		Na	sodium
KCl	potassium chloride	NB	*nota bene* (note well)
kg	kilograms	NBM	nil by mouth
kPa	kilopascals	*NEJM*	*New England Journal of Medicine*
L	left		
l	litres	NGT	nasogastric tube

NIDDM	non-insulin dependent diabetes mellitus		PRV	polycythaemia rubra vera
nocte	in the evening		PSA	prostate specific antigen
NR	normal range		PTC	percutaneous transhepatic
NSAIDs	non-steroidal anti-inflammatory drugs			cholangiography
			PTH	parathyroid hormone
O&G	obstetrics and gynaecology		PTT	prothrombin time
			PU	peptic ulcer(ation)
obs	observations		PV	*per vaginum*
OD	overdose		qds	*quarte in die somemdum* (to be taken four times a day)
od	once a day			
$Pa\text{co}_2$	partial pressure of CO_2 in arterial blood		qid	*quarte in die* (four times a day)
PAN	polyarteritis nodosa		R	right
Pap	Papanicolaou		RA	rheumatoid arthritis
$Pa\text{o}_2$	partial pressure of O_2 in arterial blood		RBBB	right bundle branch block
			RBC	red blood cell
PAYE	pay as you earn		RCC	red cell count
PBC	primary biliary cirrhosis		RF	rheumatic fever
pc	*post cibum* (after food)		Rh	rhesus
PCA	patient controlled analgesia		RTA	renal tubular acidosis/road traffic accident
PCP	*Pneumocystis carinni* pneumonia		RIF	right iliac fossa
			RS	respiratory system
PCR	polymerase chain reaction		RUQ	right upper quadrant
PCV	packed cell volume		RV	right ventricle
PE	pulmonary embolism		RVF	right ventricular failure
PEFR	peak expiratory flow rate		RVH	right ventricular hypertrophy
PID	pelvic inflammatory disease			
			Rx	treat with
PIP	proximal interphalangeal		SAH	subarachnoid haemorrhage
PM	*post mortem*			
PMH	past medical history		SBE	subacute bacterial endocarditis
PMT	premenstrual tension			
PN	percussion note		SC (sub cut)	subcutaneous
PND	paroxysmal nocturnal dyspnoea		SD	standard deviation
			SE	side effects
PO	*per orum* (by mouth)		SHO	Senior House Officer
PPD	purified protein derivative		SIADH	syndrome of inappropriate ADH secretion
PPF	purified plasma fraction			
PR	*per rectum*		SL	sublingual
PRN	*pro re nata* (as required)		SLE	systemic lupus erythematosus
pro tem	as required, on an ongoing basis			

SOA	swelling of ankles	TRH	thyrotrophin releasing
SOB	shortness of breath		hormone
SR	slow release	TSH	thyroid stimulating
SR	senior registrar		hormone
SRN	state registered nurse	TTA	to take away
SSRV	structured small round	TTO	to take out
	virus	TU	tuberculin units
stat	*statim* (immediately)	TURP	transurethral retrograde
STD	sexually transmitted		prostatectomy
	disease	TURT	transurethral retrograde
SVC	superior vena cava		tumourectomy
SVT	supraventricular	u (U)	units
	tachycardia	U&E	urea and electrolytes
SXR	skull X-ray	UC	ulcerative colitis
T	temperature	UMN	upper motorneurone
$T_{1/2}$	biological half life	URT	upper respiratory tract
T_3	triiodothyronine	US	ultrasound
T_4	thyroxine	UTI	urinary tract infection
	(tetraiodothyronine)	VF	ventricular fibrillation
TB	tuberculosis	VQ scan	ventilation perfusion
tds	*ter die somemdum* (to be		scan
	taken three times a day)	VDRL	venereal diseases research
TENS	transcutaneous electrical		laboratory
	nerve stimulation	VLDL	very low density
TG	triglyceride		lipoprotein
TIA	transient ischaemic attack	VMA (also	vanillyl-mandelic acid
TIBC	total iron binding capacity	HMMA)	
tid	*ter in die* (three times a	VSD	ventriculo-septal defect
	day)	VT	ventricular tachycardia
TLC	tender loving care	WBC	white blood cell
tPA	tissue plasminogen	WCC	white cell count
	activator	WPW	Wolff–Parkinson–White
TPN	total parenteral nutrition		syndrome
TPR	temperature, pulse and	ZN	Ziehl–Nielsen stain
	respiratory rate	Zn	zinc

Chapter 1: **Starting up**

Day one of your house job is rarely the nightmare you think it will be. Half of it is taken up by firm meetings and introductions to the hospital. During the other half you will be introduced to the wards. It's all over before you know what's happening. You are finally a real doctor. And then it's day two and you have to get on with the job . . .

Panic?

Never panic. The thing that strikes terror into the hearts of day-one House Officers is the thought that they, alone, are expected to battle with disease and death when they have never given an IV drug in their life and don't know how to plug in the paddles of the cardiac arrest trolley. That's if they know where to find it. The ward and hospital are often unfamiliar. The whole thing is enough to give you a nasty rash, which many House Officers do get.

The one thing to remember is: YOU ARE NOT ALONE. You are a modest, essential cog in a vast machine which churns away quite happily whether you know exactly what you're doing or not. You soon will. Nobody expects you to know much on the first day — or even in the first month. And everyone will show you what to do.

People to help you

You are surrounded by people who can help you. They include:
1 Nurses who usually know more about what you are doing than you do, as they have watched and done it for years.
2 Patients who are not trying to catch you out and who only want to be treated kindly, properly and with as little pain as possible.
3 Other doctors who love to demonstrate their skill at just about everything and are always open to requests for help.
• Problems arise when House Officers do NOT ask for help. If you feel panic rising in your throat, **just ask for help**. This is counter-intuitive for self-reliant medics, but it saves lives (yours and the patient's).
• Attend orientation day for House Officers if the hospital has one. It is useful for finding out what the hospital can do for you.
• If possible contact your predecessors before their last day on the job. They can give you invaluable information about what to expect from your house job (the idea for this book came from a request for help from a new House Officer). In particular, ask them about what your new consultants do and do not like.
• Most people find that they are incredibly tired during their first week of work. Such fatigue usually passes as they get used to the hospital and new routines.

Three basic tips

1 Always take initiative in hospitals. If things are not working, do something about it. Big institutions can become stupid places to work in just because no-one bothers to address things that are clearly going wrong. Figure out a solution and contact whoever is in charge of the problem, whether it be a doctor, nurse, manager or the porter.

2 Similarly, take initiative in managing patients. Present seniors with a plan for your patients rather than just asking them what to do. Thinking strategically makes patient management much more fun.

3 Order your work. When tasks are being fired at you from all directions, priority-setting is really important. Try to learn early on which things are super-urgent and which can wait for more peaceful moments. Despite the hype, there *is* quite a lot of down time in your House Officer year.

Other useful start-up information

Bibliography

Most House Officers read little other than fiction during their house-job. You probably don't need to buy anything you don't already have. A few recommended texts are:

Acute Medicine: Sprigings D. and Chambers J. (2001) Blackwell Science, Oxford. A comprehensive guide to emergencies.

Clinical Examination: Talley N. and O'-Connor S. (1996) Blackwell Science, Oxford. This book is great for revising detailed clinical examination.

Oxford Handbook of Clinical Medicine: Hope R.A. (Editor), Longmore J.M., Wood-Allum C.A., Hope T. and McManus S. (1998) Oxford University Press, Oxford. A great pocket reference text for medical and surgical conditions.

Dunn's Surgical Diagnosis and Management: A Guide to General Surgical Care: Dunn D. and Rawlinson N. (1999) Blackwell Science, Oxford. A great book for HO and SHO level surgical trainees.

The ECG Made Easy (and its sequel, *The ECG in Practice*): Hampton J. (1997) Churchill Livingstone, Edinburgh. An approachable guide to the mysteries of the ECG.

Junior Doctors' Handbook: Published annually by the BMA, free to members. An excellent summary of your rights and useful information for your early years as a doctor.

Recommended texts for the medical specialties (SHO level texts) include:

Pocket Consultant: Gastroenterology: Travis S., Taylor R. and Misiewicz J. (1998) Blackwell Science, Oxford. This book clearly explains gastroenterological problems and procedures which are invaluable for both medicine and surgery, as well as for Membership exams.

Pocket Consultant: Cardiology: Swanton R. (1998) Blackwell Science, Oxford. As for Gastroenterology above.

Lecture Notes on Respiratory Medicine: Bourke S. and Brewis R. (1998) Blackwell Science, Oxford. Beautiful explanations of the pathophysiology and principles of management of respiratory disease. A very good primer for the Chest Unit job.

Essential Neurology: Wilkinson I. (1999) Blackwell Science, Oxford. A concise and clearly illustrated guide to clinical neurology. For a more comprehensive guide to differential diagnosis consider *Patten's Neurological Differential Diagnosis* (Springer-Verlag) — a classic text.

Essential Haematology: Hoffbrand A., Pettit J and Moss P (updated every reprint; the most recent edition, 2001) Blackwell Science, Oxford. A superb book!

Essential Endocrinology: Brook C. and Marshall N. (2001) Blackwell Science, Oxford. Another very useful primer for an Endocrine Unit job.

There are no particularly good small books for rheumatology or nephrology. We recommend using the appropriate chapter in any medical textbook such as *Medicine*: Axford J. (1996) Blackwell Science or *Clinical Medicine*: Kumar and Clark (1998) Harcourt Brace, London.

Dress

It is worth bearing in mind that patients often dress up to the nines to 'visit the doctor'. I once watched an elderly woman with deteriorating eyesight, high-heeled shoes and lopsided make-up hobble over the hospital lawn to visit the diabetes clinic. Having always dressed casually, I dressed my best from then on.

• Changing from student to doctor mode can put grave dents into your early pay cheques. If nothing else, buy good quality shoes which will look good and stay comfortable on your 36th hour.

• You may get stained with all sorts of unmentionable substances as a House Officer. *Stain Devils* from supermarkets and household stores can remove most things. Soaking garments in cold water and lots of soap, followed by a normal machine wash removes blood stains.

• Most hospitals will reimburse you for dry cleaning bills associated with work-related accidents, such as major blood stains on suits. Phone hospital personnel through the switchboard.

Equipment

Always carry:
1 Pen.
2 Notebook/filofax/piece of paper.
3 Stethoscope.
4 Tourniquet.
5 Torch.
6 Bleep.
7 Loose change for food/drink/newspaper.
8 Ophthalmoscope (if not readily accessible on wards).

For ward rounds and working in casualty, as above plus:
1 White coat.
2 Tendon hammer (preferably collapsible).
3 Wooden spatula.
4 Orange sticks.

• Consider carrying everything in a traveller's pouch.

• Ensure that all equipment is labelled with your name. Hospital wrist bands are good for labelling stethoscopes. Equipment can be engraved.

• House Officers definitely need access to ophthalmoscopes. Ward ophthalmoscopes have an amazing tendency to walk and to run out of batteries. Therefore, it is advisable to acquire your own portable ophthalmoscope, and to look in people's eyes at every opportunity. Welch Allyn markets a pocket veterinary ophthalmoscope that is portable, relatively cheap and reliable, and little known to medics—as it is advertised for vets.

• Ask your ward pharmacist for a couple of aliquots of tropicamide to carry in your top pocket. One to two drops greatly facilitates ophthalmic examination. It takes a few minutes to work. Record the procedure in the notes and tell the nurse. Having failed to do the latter, I was once fast bleeped by a frantic student who thought the patient was coning. Never use tropicamide in patients with a history of glaucoma or eye surgery.

• Consider carrying a ring binder containing a handful of blood forms; radiology requests; blank drug charts; history, discharge summary and TTO sheets. Such a binder allows you to do a lot of the paperwork on ward rounds, before it gets forgotten. It also saves having to dash off to the stationery drawers in the middle of the round, which tends to go down badly with seniors.

Geography

• Get a map of the hospital from reception to help you learn where everything is.

• Specifically, find out the location of: blood gas machines, canteen, casualty, doctors' mess, drink machines, endoscopy, labs for crucial bloods, nuclear medicine, take rooms, wards, X-rays.

Ward rounds

Think of yourself as the ward round producer (much of it *is* theatre). Give yourself 15 minutes' preparation time to have everything ready. For each patient be prepared to supply:

1 Patient ID (name, age, DOA, occupation, presenting complaint).

2 Changes in condition and management since last round (with dates of change).

3 Results (any investigations carried out recently).

4 Assessment (physical, social, psychological).

5 Plan for in-patient management (future investigations, ops, drugs).

6 Plan for discharge (see p. 6).

7 X-rays (ask your seniors which ones to have available).

• Unless the patient asks for relatives to remain present, it is a generally a good idea to ask them to leave the room while the team examines the patient. Curtains are not sound proof. People will often give more information if their relatives are not present.

• Ask your registrar which X-rays to have available. Get these from the X-ray department well ahead of time (occasionally the ward clerk arranges this for you).

• Each consultant has up to five pet details that he or she wants to know about each patient. Find out what these are from your predecessor and supply them tirelessly at ward rounds (these could range from occupation to ESR to whether or not the patient has ever travelled to the tropics).

• Never say that you have done something you haven't, and never make up a result to please seniors. It is bound to backfire.

• Do not argue with colleagues in front of patients.

• Get a clear idea of the management

plan for each patient. Sometimes instructions may be dealt out in a half-hearted way, only for you to learn later (to your cost) that they were meant in earnest. Do not allow seniors to get away with this. Make definite 'action points' and if your consultant cannot be pressed into making him- or herself clear, then ask your registrar.

• If you work with a partner, such as a fellow House Officer or SHO, make sure that the jobs arising from the round are clearly allocated and meet up (say over lunch, or a cup of coffee) later in the day, to 'round up' on jobs done and tasks outstanding.

Social rounds

You need to let the social team know how your patient is going to cope (or not) on discharge.

1 Ask yourself: how is this patient going to manage physically, socially and mentally? Specifically, draw up a list of 'disabilities'. These are things that the patient *cannot do*, for whatever reason. From the Barthel Activities Index (p. 215), consider bathing, bladder, bowels, dressing, feeding, grooming, mobility, stairs, toilet, transfer.

2 Have relevant patient details ready (see below). Most are available from the medical notes and the front-page admissions sheet. Otherwise try the nurses, nursing notes, the patient, relatives and the GP.

3 If you are required to give a history, try to include the following points:
  • Patient ID.
  • Prognosis: short and long term.
  • GP and admitting rights to local hospitals (usually in the admission sheet at the front of the notes).
  • Type of residence and limitations (e.g. stairs).
  • Home support and previous reliance on social services.
  • Financial status.
  • Special problems which need to be addressed (physical, social, mental, legal).
  • Questions you want to ask members of the multidisciplinary team to help you plan for discharge of the patient.

4 Go to the meeting with specific questions you want answered. Make sure you come away with 'action points' — not just vague gestures from various team members about your patient's care (this goes for all ward rounds).

5 Translate medical jargon into normal English for social rounds, as some members of the social team may not be fully fluent in medical acronyms.

Night rounds

Always do a night round. This can mean the difference between a relatively happy house job and a sleepless nightmare. If you do nothing else, make sure you have checked off the following before going to bed:

1 Analgesia.
2 Fluids.
3 Infusions (on the few occasions where you are required to make them up, leave them in the fridge and tell the nurses where they are).
4 Sedation.
5 Sign for drugs you have verballed during the evening (p. 101).
6 Ask each team nurse on the night shift if he or she has problems that need sorting out before the morning.

• Start your night round *after* the night nurses' drug rounds have been com-

pleted. This is when they identify problems that you need to deal with before going to bed.
• Tell night staff to bleep you if they are concerned about a patient. Paradoxically, this combined with reassurance and information about worrisome patients cuts down bleeps.
• Inform every team nurse of what to do if a sick patient's condition changes. Sometimes you can set limits for relevant signs (e.g. pulse, CVP, T, BP) beyond which you want to be called. Write these in the notes.
• If bleeped for an apparently trivial matter, try your best not to sound irritated. Be ready to go to the ward, even if only to provide reassurance. Again, paradoxically, this reduces bleeps. If nurses are confident that you will turn up if requested, they will not bleep you ahead of time.
• If your room is a long way from the wards, you can sleep in a side room on the ward. Ask the sister or charge nurse, who will usually oblige, especially if you offer to strip the sheets in the morning. Point out that you are more readily available if you are sleeping on the ward. You might get brought cups of tea and breakfast in bed!

Discharging patients

Clearing hospital beds is an invaluable skill which will earn you lots of brownie points from virtually everyone. To clear beds effectively:
1 Make plans for people's discharge on the day they arrive. Ask yourself:
  • When will they be likely to leave?
  • What will get in the way of this person going home or being transferred?

• What can be followed up in clinic?
2 If possible, write discharge summaries (see p. 13) the day *before* the patient leaves to avoid delays.

Work environment

Evidence suggests that upgrading your environment upgrades your work — and you. Old, decrepit NHS hospitals can be rather depressing. There are ways you can make your particular corner of it a great place to work, even if the rest of the hospital has miles of yellow peeling paint, dripping pipes and corridors of empty wards.
• There is no crime in asking hospital supplies for better furniture and accessories, like shelving, desk, chairs or bulletin boards. They can always say no.
• Take a plant to work.
• If you have a tiny desk (or no desk), order a better one. Ring hospital supplies and ask if there is a spare one somewhere. Or request a new one. There's nothing like drawers that slide open easily for making paperwork easy. As a doctor with tons of notes to write, you are entitled to a desk of some kind.
• Consider buying a cheap tape deck for your desk ± earphones. Label it clearly with 'Dr X' — ours have never been stolen. It can do wonders for long winter weekends and nights on call.
• Put postcards/pictures/photos up in your work area. If you don't have a bulletin board, order one from hospital supplies.
• Buy/borrow/beg a spare typewriter if you like writing. In one of my house jobs I had my typewriter permanently on my desk. It made form-filling a lot easier, and enabled me to write letters and

stories when I was bored out of my brain on weekend cover.

• Bring decent coffee or cocoa supplies to work. A single-cup cafetiere, some packs of coffee at the back of the ward fridge and jar of your favourite spread can upgrade your existence no end.

• If your ward has photos of the 'ward team' on it, ring Medical Illustration and get them to take photos of the doctors on the ward and put them up too.

Chapter 2: **Getting organized (four lists and a folder)**

Keeping track of patients and their details can be the bane of your life as an House Officer. Filling in forms after work is a waste of precious evenings. Fortunately, you can greatly reduce the time you spend chasing paper, patients and results by having four lists and a folder.

Personal folder

A ring binder folder can save days of time on ward rounds and on night call. Unlike a filofax, a folder provides a writing surface at the bedside and an immediate supply of forms during ward rounds, so that you can do all the paperwork during rounds and don't have to return to the ward later. As well as saving time, using a folder means you are less likely to forget things, because you can do most tasks as soon as they are requested.

How to make a personal folder:

1 You need one A4 ring binder folder with a large plastic pocket inside the front cover, and at least two sets of brightly coloured dividers (WH Smith sells them cheaply).

2 Fill the folder with all the different forms you use during the day, stacking each type of form behind different dividers. Label the dividers. Stuff small forms (e.g. blood forms) in the inside pocket. Useful forms include:

Accident forms, blood cards (biochemistry, haematology, bacteriology), consent forms, CT cards, discharge forms, drug charts, ECG forms, firm timetable, fluid charts, history sheets, nuclear medicine cards, X-ray forms.

3 If forms are not already hole-punched, you can almost always find a hole-puncher at the ward clerk's desk.

4 Consider sticking a page of phone numbers and/or drug regimens (see p. 9) to the front of your folder for easy reference.

Keeping track of patients (List 1)

This is a hassle. People have devised many complex strategies for ensuring that they have up-to-date details for each patient. However you do it, you need information to hand so that you can answer questions on ward rounds, discuss patients over the phone with GPs, nurses and colleagues, write in the notes and do the discharge summary, and request and find results of investigations. The minimum information for this includes:

• Patient name and hospital number.
• Reason for admission and major details from PMH.
• Main problems now.
• Mainstay of management (e.g. drugs, surgery).
• Recent results.

One way of keeping track of such information is to stick patient labels onto history sheets, leaving a space between

Name	Extension	Name	Extension
Anaesthetist		Microbiology	
Bereavement officer		Microbiology on-call	
Biochem		MRI	
Biochem on-call		Nurses' room	
Blood transfusion		OT	
Casualty		Outpatients	
Clotting lab		Pain clinic	
Consultant secretary		Pathology	
CT		Personnel	
Cytopathology		Pharmacist	
Day hospital		Pharmacy-dispensary	
Dermatology referral		Physiotherapy	
Diabetic clinic		Porters	
Doctors' mess		Post mortems	
Doctors' residence		Pulmonary function	
Doctors' room		Records	
Drug information		Registrar	
ECG		Security	
Echo		SHO	
Endoscopy		Social workers	
Gastro referral		SR	
Gerontology referral		Stoma nurse	
Haematology		Take-away	
Haematology on-call		Theatre-reception	
Immunology		Theatre-recovery	
Infection control		Ultrasound	
Library		Wards	
Linen		X-ray	
Librarian		X-ray (portable)	
Medical records			

Fig. 2.1 Essential telephone numbers.

each to fill in patient details. Put a line
through patients who have been dis-
charged. The labels contain patient ID.
A sheet like this can be made up as
patients are admitted in casualty, and
stored at the front of a personal folder.

List of things to do (List 2)

The simplest ways to keep track of many
tasks are to:
1 Keep a daily list on the back of a card
that you can update regularly.
2 Keep a small diary to note down
requests for days and weeks ahead.
• Write down all requests as soon as you
receive them.
• Try subdividing tasks in terms of
where they have to be done. This enables
you to choreograph your movements
around the hospital rather than endlessly
dashing from one ward to another. For
example:

X-ray	give in forms from ward round
	ask Dr A about Mr B's CT
	request barium enema for Mr C
Ward 6A	IV line for Mrs D
	consent Mr E for colon-oscopy

Ward 7B	vitamin K for Ms F
	sign verbal for paracetamol

Phone numbers (List 3)

Phone numbers are essential. Making a
list early saves a lot of time. You can
reduce the list with a photocopier and
stick it on the front of your filofax or
ward folder for easy reference. From
experience, it is easier to find names if
the list is strictly alphabetical. Copy or
modify Fig. 2.1 if you like.

Firm timetable (List 4)

Hospitals have their own days for doing
speciality procedures (such as isotope
scans). Colleagues and relevant departments will know what these are.

Get a copy of your team's timetable.
Find out from your colleagues what you
need to bring for team activities such
as X-ray conferences and academic
meetings.

Chapter 3: **Paperwork**

Paperwork is not difficult—just boring. As doctors communicate with many people through forms and notes, it is important that they contain clear information. The most important part of paperwork is writing clear, legible patient notes.

Patient notes

Doctors are legally obliged to write in patients' notes at least once every third day. However, it is good practice to write something every day.

1 Always sign notes and print your surname clearly with your bleep number.

2 It is useful to ask two things when writing patient notes:
- Do the notes give enough information to treat the patient when I'm not available?
- Will I be legally covered if these notes were ever before a court?

3 For daily notes, try this checklist (CRAP):

C hange in the patient's condition or management.

R esults of investigations (blood, X-ray and otherwise).

A ssessment of patient's physical and psychological states.

P lan for future (management and discharge).

(SOAP (Subjective, Objective, Assessment, Plan) is another popular acronym. Choose whichever you prefer.)

4 If you're not sure about how to document a patient's condition, flick back through previous notes and see how others approached it—or ask a colleague.

5 It is helpful for subsequent readers if you include the time, date and place (e.g. casualty) in the margin of notes.

6 If you are called to see a patient, briefly document (even if the call was trivial):
- That you saw the patient.
- The time and date.

7 It is foolhardy to write anything in the notes that you would not want the patient or their relatives to read; they have legal access to them.

8 It is perfectly admissible to write 'no change' or words to that effect if nothing much has happened to the patient.

9 Writing how the patient seems to you (e.g. cheerful, sad, fed up) gives a good baseline for future management.

Accident forms

When called to see a patient who has had an accident (e.g. fell out of bed):

1 See the patient as soon as possible. Nurses are legally liable unless they make sure you see the patient.

2 Ask the patient what happened and which part hurts the most. Check:
- T, BP, pulse and respiratory rate.
- Consciousness level (see Glasgow Coma Scale, p. 216).
- Skin for bruising, bleeding, cuts and fractures.

• Bone tenderness and shape for fractures. Frail patients can sustain fractures with remarkably little fuss. Especially look for hip, wrist and scaphoid fractures. Examine the skull carefully if the patient hits his or her head. Consult with your senior if there is sign of serious injury or drowsiness—he or she may request a CT or skull X-ray (see pp. 180 & 183).

3 Sign an accident form (the nurses will give you one). Filling it in is self-explanatory.

4 Also write in patient's notes. Include:
• Time and date.
• Brief history of accident.
• Brief examination findings.
• That you signed an accident form.

5 If appropriate, ask the nurses to continue observations at regular intervals and to contact you if the patient's condition deteriorates.

6 Think about how the accident occurred. If possible, make a plan with the nurses to prevent future accidents.

7 Consider carrying a couple of accident forms in a personal folder (see p. 8); it saves time in the middle of the night.

Blood forms and requesting bloods

• Ask haematologists and biochemists which details on blood cards are essential. Often the cards have spaces for information that is unnecessary.

• Write your bleep and ward number clearly on blood cards so the labs can contact you if necessary.

• Two good times to fill in forms are during the daily ward round and when writing in patients' notes. Having a stack of forms ready saves time.

• Where possible, anticipate patients'

Table 3.1 Conditions for which it may be possible to fill out serial forms.

MI on admission	Lipids (only worth doing within 12 hours of infarct; values will change post-MI for 3 months)
Days 1–3	Serial cardiac enzymes
	Serial ECGs
Warfarin initiation	Check the INR at least:
	Every day for 1 week
	Every week for 3 weeks
	Every month for 3 months
	Every 8 weeks after that
Renal failure: daily	C&E, Urea
TPN: daily	C&E
Mon, Wed, Fri	LFTs, Ca, phosphate, alkaline phosphatase
Weekly	Mg, Zn, FBC, urea
IV fluids: daily	C&E, urea
Post-op bloods: next day	C&E
	FBC, urea

blood needs and write forms in bulk. For example, if someone has had a suspected MI, you can write out a stack of cardiac enzyme forms on admission, or on the ward round the next day, for 3 days. Conditions for which it is sometimes possible to fill in serial forms include those shown in Table 3.1.

• Try having a separate plastic bag or a hook or paper clamp for each day of the week in the doctors' office. You can write serial forms at the start of the week and see at a glance who needs what. Alternatively you can stack forms in chronological order on a clipboard.

• One way of keeping track of patients' tests is to write 'FBC' (or whatever) and date under the patient's label in your list of patient details (p. 8).

• If you don't have a phlebotomist, don't despair. Taking bloods in the morning enables you to sort out patients' problems before the ward round and enables you to say good morning to patients on a one-on-one basis. This has remarkable effects on one's efficacy.

Consent (see p. 189)

Death and cremation certificates (see pp. 95, 97)

Discharge summaries (TTO/TTA) (also see Discharging patients, p. 6)

The discharge summary or 'TTO' or 'TTA' (To Take Out or Away) is a sheet that House Officers write for patients to take to their GPs. It enables GPs to continue with outpatient care until the more detailed discharge letter arrives. The letter is usually written by the SHO or registrar but may fall to you. The TTO is also the prescription form that the nurses use to order drugs for patients to take home with them (although some hospitals provide a separate form for this function).

1 Get the GP's name and address from the patient or the front page of the notes.
2 Complete the TTO before the patient leaves! Include:
  • Patient details.
  • Name of consultant.
  • Name of ward.
  • Diagnosis.
  • Important findings, positive and negative.
  • Treatment given.
  • Treatment on discharge.
  • Follow-up arrangements.
  • What the patient has been told.
  • Your name and bleep number.
3 Patients are often delayed in hospital because TTOs have not been written. Write them as soon as possible so that drugs can be fetched from pharmacy. Patients and nurses will love you for this.
4 Carry a bunch of TTOs on ward rounds so that you can write the TTO on the spot when the decision is made to send someone home. This means that you can check any discharge details with the team, and the form can be sent to pharmacy pronto.
5 Phone the GP on discharge if the patient:
  • Self-discharges.
  • Is in an unstable condition.
  • Has poor home circumstances.
  • Dies.
  • Needs an early visit.
6 Consider phoning the GP if you are discharging a patient with particularly

complex or sensitive care needs, such as elderly people living alone or terminally ill patients.

Drug charts (see p. 99)

Drug prescriptions (see p. 100)

Handovers

Before you go home, to bed or away for the weekend you will need to 'hand over' your patients to the doctor who replaces you. This can usually be done over the phone or a quick coffee. Obviously how much detail you tell your successor depends on whether or not they are familiar with the patients—bear in mind that they may not know them at all. You need to make sure your successors know:
1 Who your patients are, which ward they are on and why they are in hospital.
2 A brief summary of the management of each patient (e.g. awaiting surgery tomorrow, NBM, needs continuous morphine infusion for pain relief but stable).
3 Likely complications or difficulties and how you have been dealing with these to date.
4 Anyone (doctor/nurse/relatives) who may be contacted if problems arise.
5 If you are handing over to a locum who is new to the hospital, you will help him or her enormously by spending a few minutes sharing key information about the layout of the hospital and how to perform routine tasks (see Locums, p. 206).

Hand backs

It is common to 'hand back' patients to consultants who have looked after them within the last 1–2 years, but check your hospital's policy. It is helpful to hand back patients early in the day to give the accepting team a fair chance to assess the patient themselves. It is good practice to make sure that investigations suggested on the post-take round have been completed prior to the hand back. The accepting doctor should be aware of any outstanding tests and the admitting team's provisional diagnosis. Don't forget to explain to the patient what is happening!

Referral letters

If you need to refer a patient to another team, you can either phone the registrar of that team and leave relevant details in the patient's notes, or write the consultant a letter, or both. If you write a letter, include the following:
1 Address the letter to the consultant of the other team.
2 Name of your consultant, yourself and your bleep number.
3 Name of patient, age, sex, DOB, hospital ID and current location (e.g. ward/home).
4 Name of patient's GP.
5 Specific question(s) your team needs answered.
6 Relevant clinical history and examination findings.
7 Recent investigations (including negatives).
8 When you need his or her advice by.
Try to anticipate which investigations

the other team might need, and have them ready. For example, surgeons almost always need a recent FBC and maybe an ECG if they are considering theatre. Gastroenterologists, or any specialist doing a biopsy, will want an INR if investigating liver complaints. See pp. 127–132 for a list of investigations that different specialists are likely to need.

Self-discharge

However it may feel, hospitals are not prisons. Unless patients seem likely to incur life-threatening harm to themselves, you cannot restrain them from leaving hospital (even when it is patently idiotic for them to do so). If your patient decides to leave against your advice, try the following:

• Explain to them why they should stay.
• Inform your senior.
• Have the patient sign a self-discharge note. This is usually available from the ward clerk. If necessary, you can write one yourself. It is a good idea to have a second witness to sign the note:

I, (*Jo Bloggs*) hereby state that I am leaving (*Name of Hospital*) against medical advice on (*today's date*). Witnessed by Dr (*Your surname*), (*today's date*) and (*Colleague's name, today's date*)
(*Jo Bloggs's signature*)
(Your name and signature)
(Second witness name and signature)

• Rarely, you may consider using the Mental Health Act to section a patient and restrain them from leaving. Always seek senior advice before doing this (p. 216).
• Make a brief note of what happened in the patient's notes.
• Inform the patient's GP that the patient has self-discharged.

Sick notes

You may be asked to write a sick note for patients to verify that they have been unable to work. There are two types of sick notes you can write:

1 If the patient is *not* trying to claim state benefit, they need a hand-written note on hospital-headed paper. The easiest way to address it is 'To Whom It May Concern' along the top, followed by something like: 'Mrs A has been an inpatient at the X Hospital from 24–30 April and will be unable to return to work until May 7'. Sign and date it, and block print your name and position under your signature as well as the name of the patient's consultant.

In this kind of letter, you should *not* disclose the patient's condition. If in doubt, ask your senior.

2 If the patient *is* trying to claim state benefit after leaving hospital, they need a **Med 3** form to be signed by you (ask your ward clerk, registrar or phone the nearest DSS office). This is self-explanatory, but you must fill in the diagnosis. Ask your senior if you have any doubts about it.

Chapter 4: **Accident and emergency**

Working shifts in A&E can be a lot of fun, or it can result in the weekend from hell, working 'til you drop. As usual, being organized and armed with a few hints makes a big difference to coping well.

General

During both medical and surgical takes you see the same handful of conditions most of the time (see below). Whatever your baseline knowledge, you soon become adept at treating them.

• Do not be afraid to ask nurses for advice. They have seen it all before.

• You can spend a lot of time looking for equipment in casualty. Try preparing batches of forms and bottles when things are quiet. Suggested forms include (per patient):

2 history sheets, drug chart, fluid chart, X-ray form, blood cards, consent form.

• Try equipping yourself with a metal trolley at the beginning of the shift. It helps to keep your equipment in one place and gives you a surface to work on.

• Try sticking a yellow plastic bag to the edge of the trolley for rubbish; it saves trips to the garbage with packaging. A small yellow sharps bin is ideal if you can find one.

• Tape two or three sheets of paper to your 'take' desk. Use these to note down accepted patients, so as not to lose track

of expected (and received) patients. These sheets can also be used to document tentative and confirmed diagnoses, the results of initial tests, and the ward to which the patient is sent from casualty. You can then use the sheets to lead the post-take round.

• Dehydration is a real problem if you work without a break in casualty. Suggest to the medical or surgical hospital manager that a drinking water dispenser be installed in casualty. Drink as many fluids as you can.

• Take meal breaks ruthlessly. Hold the fort for your colleagues and have them do the same for you. No-one works efficiently with hypoglycaemia.

• It is easier to move in casualty without a white coat. This is possible even if you wear a pocketless skirt or trousers; clip pens and bleep to your waistband. Alternatively wear a travel pouch.

Admitting and allocating patients

1 Ask medical and nursing colleagues about the local routine for admitting and allocating patients during take.
2 When a GP telephones you to admit a patient:
• Be polite.
• Have paper and pen ready.
• Listen first.
• Take down: Name.
Age.
Problem.

Hospital number.
GP name and number.
When to expect the
    patient's arrival.
• Phone casualty or the ward with the patient's details.
• Let your senior know that the patient is coming in and their main complaint.

3 If you accept a patient from a GP, then you are obliged to clerk them, even if it is obvious that they need to be transferred to another specialty. Try, therefore, to transfer the call to the right specialist *before* the patient arrives, or you will end up seeing the patient, however inappropriately.

4 You may bear the brunt of poor bed allocation. Consider negotiating with admissions, the managing sister or charge nurse ('bed manager') and clinical managers to work out a better system. It helps to know the wards' bed status when working in A&E, so you can send patients where you want them.

Keeping track of patients

• Whatever you do, get results for patients before you go to bed and make sure you have them ready for the post-take ward round.
• Try keeping a history sheet with patient stickers down one side with results of baseline tests and a thumbnail sketch of the main problems on each sticker. This is invaluable for post-take ward rounds.
• If you are missing results, check the casualty result book before retiring.
• If you urgently need a result after midnight, you can usually get recent results from the technician's book in the lab.

There is usually a duty biochemist or haematologist on call.

Medicine

On admission, try to complete for each medical patient:

1 History and examination.
2 Baseline tests: FBC, C&E, glucose,
                        ESR, CRP
                    MSU and dipstick
                    ECG
                    CXR (consider erect
                        CXR if suspected
                        perforation)
                    Consider clotting
                        screen
                        (INR/KCCT),
                        LFTs
3 IV access.
4 Fluid chart for 24 hours.
5 Drug chart.

The most common medical emergencies
1 Haematemesis (peptic ulcer or gastritis)
2 Unstable angina
3 MI
4 Stroke (infarct or haemorrhagic)
5 DVT and PE
6 'Off legs' or collapse
7 Overdose

Overdose

Medical House Officers see many patients who have overdosed. A&E get the slashed wrists and other forms of bodily mutilation, but you have to deal with people's gastric contents. Do not panic with overdose patients. There is usually more time than you realize to sort them out and the vast majority do not take devastating overdoses. You can (and should) get senior medical and nursing assistance if the patient *is* in a critical condition. They may need transfer to ITU. Never wash out an uncooperative or unconscious patient without the supervision of an anaesthetist.

In general

• If in **any** doubt about how to treat someone, phone the 24-hour Poisons hotline (switchboard and A&E staff will have these numbers). Their staff will tell you exactly what to do, according to your patient's symptoms and history.

Poisons information
Belfast 028 9024 0503
Birmingham 0121 507 5588
0121 507 5589
Cardiff 029 2070 9901
Dublin 00353 1 837 9964
00353 1 837 9966
Edinburgh 0131 536 2300
London 020 7635 9191
Newcastle 0191 282 0300

• The *BNF* has an excellent section on treatments for different substance overdoses at the beginning of the book (look under 'Poison' in the index). We have not tried to replicate the *BNF* information here, as it is more detailed and up to date in the *BNF* itself.

Treating the patient

First, briefly assess the patient

1 If the patient is unconscious, seek senior help. Make sure the unconscious patient is in the coma position and check the airway for tongue, dentures or vomit.
2 If the patient is drowsy or unconscious, alert an anaesthetist to intubate the patient for a washout. Get senior advice. The patient may need to be transferred to ITU.
3 Quickly check for and treat hypoxia, hypotension and hypovolaemia (from vomiting and tachypnoea), hypoglycaemia, hypothermia and arrhythmias. Ask the nurses to do a blood glucose stick, ECG, BP and pulse oximeter reading, particularly if the patient is semi-conscious. Consider doing a blood gas and rectal temperature.
4 Secure IV access. Consider immediate, rapid IV fluid if the patient is in shock.
5 Take the following samples from the patient:
    Biochemistry sample:
        C&E, urea, LFTs, salicylate and paracetamol levels. These need repeating if less than 4 hours have elapsed since the overdose
    Glucose sample
        (liver damage causes hypoglycaemia)
    Serum sample (at least one)
        Storage—in case there is need to do further tests
    INR (acute liver failure will cause a rising prothrombin time)
    Sample of vomitus (to biochemistry)
        Label with time, date and suspected substance

It is standard practice to check drug levels (principally salicylate and paracetamol) for all overdose patients. Patients may conceal or simply not realize how many tablets they have taken, or whether they contain these substances. Paracetamol levels should be taken not less than 4 hours after ingestion, aspirin not less than 6 hours, but longer if the tablets have enteric coating.

• Always collect at least one sample of blood from the patient, regardless of what they claim to have taken.

• Lethal paracetamol overdoses may not become apparent for several days, when the person starts to go yellow. **Always assume that the person has taken paracetamol, and more than they say they have.** The Parvolex treatment chart found in A&E (see Fig. 4.1) is used to assess whether or not the patient needs treatment with a Parvolex infusion (acetylcysteine — see the *BNF* for dosage) to counteract a paracetamol overdose. Take blood levels at least 4 hours (but less than 8) after the patient has ingested the tablets.

If the level is *on or above* the line, the patient needs urgent treatment or risks fatal liver damage. Be prepared for potentially serious side effects, including bronchospasm, hypoglycaemia, shock and vomiting. Glucose should be checked hourly. Patients may not be sure when they took the overdose. Newer guidelines suggest erring on the side of treatment if uncertain. However, if you feel unsure about whether to treat or not, get senior advice quickly.

Levels *below* the line do not usually require treatment unless the patient has existing liver damage or is taking enzyme-inducing drugs such as carba-

mazepine. Consult with your senior. Levels need to be rechecked to make sure that they are not rising.

Aspirin overdose causes metabolic acidosis, so consider monitoring arterial blood gases. Symptoms and signs include tachypnoea, tachycardia and tinnitus.

Second, decide if the patient needs to be washed out

Washouts (gastric lavage)

NEVER wash out an unconscious patient without first intubating the patient with an anaesthetist's assistance. Consider washing patients out within:

   4 hours for anything except corrosive agents and petrol.

   6 hours for opiates and anticholinergics.

   12 hours for salicylates, aminophylline, tricyclic antidepressants.

• Ask someone to show you how to do your first few washouts. Believe it or not, you will soon get used to it!

• Gum boots and a plastic apron save your clothes during washouts.

• Be sure to use *warm* water to wash the patient out. Cold water is painful and may induce angina.

• Coat the hosepipe with lubricant jelly before insertion; it makes it much easier to swallow.

• Do not forget to follow the water washout with a bottle of charcoal solution to prevent further absorption.

• Save a specimen jar of vomitus for biochemical analysis.

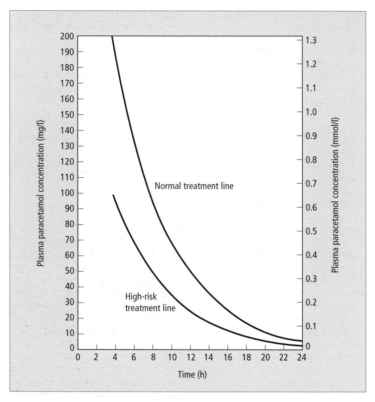

Fig 4.1 Chart to decide who should receive Parvolex. (Reproduced with kind permission of Department of Analytical Toxicology, University of Wales College of Medicine.) People at or above the treatment lines should receive treatment in accordance with guidelines published in the *British National Formulary*, providing they have no contra-indications.

Patients refusing treatment

You *can* section someone who refuses to be treated (see p. 216) if you think they have taken something that may be lethal. Obviously use this as a last resort. Sec-tioning someone is a complex process and may have serious consequences for them. Get senior advice. Sometimes when faced with the prospect of being sectioned, patients change their mind about being washed out.

**Third, do a more thorough history
and examination**

1 If possible, get a thorough history
from the patient *as well as* from whoever
accompanied them to hospital. If possible, try to ascertain:

A What precipitated the attempt?

• Intention at time of overdose (did
they mean to kill themselves?)

• Previous intentions (have they felt
like this often?)

• Was the attempt impulsive or
premeditated?

• Did they try to avoid being found?

• Did they leave a note?

• Did the patient take illicit drugs
or alcohol?

• Did the patient have specific
problems that caused them to consider suicide?

B How likely are they to try to kill themselves again?

• How do they feel about being alive?

• Do they still want to die?

• Psychiatric disorder, especially
depressive disorders with insomnia,
anorexia and weight loss

• Chronic/serious physical disorder

• Alcohol dependence

• Social isolation

• Unemployment

• Male

• >50 years old

2 Examine the patient thoroughly.

3 Perform a mini-mental test score (see
p 217).

**Fourth, discuss the patient with
your senior if you haven't already:
you will probably need to refer the
patient to the psychiatrists**

Surgery

On admission, try to complete:

1 History and examination.

2 Baseline tests: FBC, C&E, glucose,
amylase, G&S or
cross-match
MSU & dipstick,
consider
pregnancy test
ECG
AXR, consider erect
CXR

3 IV access.

4 Fluid chart for 24 hours.

5 Consent.

6 Drug chart.

• It is cruel to leave patients in acute
pain. Ambulance staff and nurses cannot
give pain relief until a doctor has seen
them. If someone has renal colic, for
example, you may be able to diagnose
this quickly and prescribe analgesia
accordingly.

• Diclofenac sodium (Voltarol) provides
effective pain relief for renal colic. It can
be given IM or by suppository.

• Very occasionally, patients who are
seeking opiates *or* a stay in hospital may
fake surgical conditions. Look for needle
marks, small pupils and odd histories. If
you suspect a patient is faking pain, ask
for senior advice. It is extremely dodgy
to 'punish' addict patients (or anyone
else) with insufficient pain relief. If your
patient is an opiate addict *and* has a real
surgical condition, then they will need
extra relief for severe pain.

Most common conditions for surgical emergency admissions

1 Acute abdomen (appendicitis and other RIF pain, UTI, obstruction, IBD, IBS)

• Always be aware of the possibility of pregnancy or gynaecological conditions in young women with abdominal pain. It is routine to request pregnancy tests on urine specimens

2 Renal colic

3 Changing catheters

• Urological conditions, such as changing catheters, renal colic, haematuria, can sometimes be referred to the urologists

Chapter 5: **Becoming a better doctor**

Postgraduate medical education used to be fairly limited, to the detriment of doctors' morale and brain cells. Fortunately, 'Continuing Medical Education' is rapidly improving through the postgraduate colleges. There are many things you can do to keep your work interesting and to prevent the whisky bottle from becoming too attractive.

Computers (if you are already a PC hack, skip this section!)

We recommend becoming as computer literate as possible, because so much medical information and worldwide communication is becoming available through the Internet (see below). If it's any consolation, our nearest and dearest relatives who recently shrieked in horror at the thought of booting up are now happily e-mailing each other, surfing merrily, and doing their banking and accounts using home PCs.

Inevitably, what we write in this section today will seem archaic by next week. Things move fast, but don't feel unnerved.

Hardware (i.e. the computer itself): what to buy?

Computer prices are falling rapidly. If you can afford it, it is probably advisable to buy a more advanced machine that you will be happy with for several years and which will keep up with increasingly sophisticated software. We strongly recommend consulting a recent computing magazine for articles that compare different brands and models.

• At the time this manuscript was written, a decent personal computer (either laptop or desk-top model) is an 800 MHz or faster Pentium III with 128 Mb RAM, and at least 6.0 Gb HDD (Hard Disk Drive) memory. As databases and journals are increasingly going on-line and becoming available on CD-ROM, it is probably a good idea to buy a package that includes an internal **modem,** and a CD-ROM drive.

• The powerful 'iMac' *Apple Macintosh* computers are now relatively price-competitive with the major PC brands, for similar computing power, although PC clones are usually cheaper. Similar specifications for *Apple* computers apply. The *iMac* models can translate and use most PC software.

• Make sure that you have a good service and parts warranty for your computer. Ideally, the company will supply an 'on-site' service and parts warranty, which means that it will send a representative to your home for a specified period of time, free of charge, if anything goes wrong.

• Check which software packages come with the computer. Some deals include tons of great software, including full word processing, spreadsheet and graphics programs. You will pay a lot if you have to buy all this yourself.

• When ordering your computer, check

the available date of delivery If you have to wait 3 months, switch firms!

• One good way to buy a computer is to order it directly from the manufacturer, rather than going through a retailer. The (usually toll-free) numbers of companies can be found in the *Yellow Pages* and in any major computing magazine.

• Find out from your consultant or BMA office if there is any way you can claim an educational discount (or if the health authority could help you pay for the computer) on the grounds that it helps you with NHS work. Consider claiming it as a tax deduction.

• In addition to magazine consumer surveys, try tracking down the person who maintains and buys computers for your hospital. They may be able to guide you in purchasing a computer.

• Consider buying a lap-top computer, which is much more convenient for the mobile junior doctor. You can always buy a large screen and keyboard to plug into the lap-top if you want to make it easier to use at home.

• A palm-held computer may be useful for the wards as well as your personal life. Palm-held computers provide a limited number of applications, like personal organizers, directories, word processors and spreadsheets. They may be synchronized with your lap-top or desk-top and act as a portable extension of your computer. An increasing amount of software is becoming available for palm-helds, including applications designed for patient management. Make sure your PC can support the software and hardware needed to link to a palm-held computer before going out and buying one.

• If you need to buy a monitor, for enhanced quality of life treat yourself to a 15″ or larger screen (rather than the regular 14″ screen). Bear in mind also that you can buy ergonomic keyboards and mice that can really improve your comfort level if you use the computer a lot.

Software

There are so many different brands of software with a myriad of functions. We suggest that you consider the following generic types of software programs to help organize your files and save you oodles of time while making your work look professional.

1 Word processing package (e.g. Microsoft Word, WordPerfect). It is possible to convert *MS Word* files to *WordPerfect* files and vice versa so it is really a matter of institutional preference which you use. MS Word is more widely used within medicine.

2 Bibliographic database package (e.g. *Idealist*, *Procite*, *Reference Manager*). These programs are great if you are interested in keeping long-term files or notes on just about anything. Basically, they enable you to write notes and bibliographic references on whatever you want (such as journal articles and talks you've been to) and then recall any text or reference word with a few key strokes. They are a good way of beating the paper tiger into submission.

3 Slide and overhead presentation package (e.g. *Powerpoint*)—enables you to make professional-looking slides and overheads.

4 Spreadsheet program (e.g. *Excel*, *Lotus*) enables you to do accounts and present tabulated, quantitative data.

5 Communications software. Most modern machines are 'Internet-ready' straight out of the box, so you probably

will not need to worry about this unless you are souping-up an old computer.

6 Desk-top publishing software (e.g. *PageMaker*) enables you to produce professional-looking newsletters/publications.

7 Virus detection software will prevent your files and computer from being 'infected' with destructive computer viruses.

Other ways of getting access to on-line databases

There are now many websites offering free access to MEDLINE. We recommend PubMed (http://www.ncbi.nlm.nih.gov/PubMed) as it has a user-friendly search engine that offers free access to medline. Increasingly, hospital and university libraries have on-line databases available over the Internet. There are numerous medical information providers, although quality control is the major problem with most. The TRIPS database is a free, quality-controlled medical search engine, available at http://www.tripdatabase.com. A number of journals are now provided free on the web, and most will allow you to read archived abstracts from papers in back issues, and to contribute to on-line discussion. Some even allow you to read the full text from back issues, all absolutely free, e.g. *BMJ* (http://www.bmj.com), *JAMA* (http://www.jama.com).

A bit about the Internet

Modems are essential because they enable you to access the Internet and the rapidly expanding world of internation-al information networks. Why is this so important? We (and lots of others) believe that the world is undergoing something of another technological revolution in which rapid information exchange is transforming the way people live and work. Learning how to access this information will keep you from becoming scared of it—and give you an enormous advantage in your work.

The Internet is a vast, sprawling electronic network, which extends as far as there are phone lines (or satellites). It was originally set up by the US military to improve communication between international military stations, but since then it has been somewhat swamped by millions of other users world-wide. The Internet enables individuals from every part of the globe to talk to one another via their computers within seconds, and to tap into whatever information sources lie at the end of the millions of lines.

To tap into the Internet you need to be connected to a local 'node'. Tapping in may cost you money, unless you can connect through a hospital or university that has free access to the Internet (some do and some don't—ask your hospital computer person). Check out the different Internet service providers, and see which is the best deal for your pattern of usage. Some make no flat monthly charge, but you still have to pay for using the phone line (just as if you were making a phone call), although this is usually, but not always, at local rates. Others charge a flat rate, and allow you a fixed amount of free connection time. Even after you have signed up, you can swap to a different provider, should you find a better deal. It may not be long before web access is absolutely free of charge. Hospital libraries and departments usually offer free Internet access 24 hours a day, although you may have to book a slot on the library computers to use the service.

We won't wax lyrical here about all the things you can access over the 'Net'. There are many user-friendly books on this subject in most large book-stores. Medical journals are increasingly advertising databases and users' bulletin boards which can be accessed through the Net and the World Wide Web (WWW). The web can provide access to a myriad of evidence-based resources and also provide news, views and services specifically for young doctors, although you have to know where to look and how to sort the wheat from the chaff. It is probably worth signing up with one of the free portals for doctors, such as http://www.doctors.net.uk, http://www.medix.co.uk, or www.medicsworld.com to help you navigate and to ease you in to the on-line community.

How to access the Internet

1 Your computer is most likely to contain an internal modem already. If not, buy and install an external modem and accompanying communications software package (get help with this from your computer store or hospital computer person).

2 Establish with a local university or hospital how to 'dial in' to their Internet node, or subscribe to an Internet service provider, which will enable you to access the Internet.

3 Buy or borrow a book about the Internet so that you don't miss out on the tons of information highways/bulletin boards/public information available.

Keeping up with the literature

The information and technology explosion is very real. There are currently over 25 000 biomedical journals in print, and this figure is rising exponentially.* How on earth can you keep up with the literature?

Actually, you can. There are several great ways to keep up to date with stacks of international journals with minimal fuss (we wish we knew about these when we were students):

• Invest in a personal computer and bibliographic software package (see p. 24). These allow you to make superquick notes and references of good things you read or hear so that you can access them years from now. Say goodbye to bulging filing cabinets and disorganized papers and build your own personal database which will serve you for talks, presentations and your own interests for the rest of your professional life.

• Adopt a 'problem-based' approach to reading. This means reading whatever you need to answer real questions, rather than blindly scanning journals with minimal retention and maximum boredom (see Evidence-based medicine, below). You will remember much more of what you read if your patient depends upon it and you'll probably also find it more interesting.

• If you *do* want to scan scientific studies, try reading the *BMJ*'s bimonthly journal, *Evidence-Based Medicine*, which contains critically appraised summaries of the most recent, good

---

* Wyatt J. (1991) Uses and sources of medical knowledge. *Lancet* **338**, 1368–1373.

quality medical trials articles from a wide range of international journals.
• Read review articles before you read other kinds of studies. Good quality systematic reviews, especially those using meta-analysis, are the most efficient studies to read* because they combine the results of many individual studies, adding statistical power and giving you an efficient overview of the topic. The *BMJ's Clinical Evidence* is a fabulous resource, published every 6 months and available on-line at www.evidence.org. It is an ever-expanding directory of question-driven systematic reviews about treatments. It will even tell you when there is no good quality literature about a topic. The Cochrane Library (CL) contains both the Cochrane Collaboration and NHS Centre for Reviews and Dissemination's databases of systematic reviews. The CL is currently being installed on hospital computers throughout the UK, and *Clinical Evidence* will now be provided free by the UK government to all UK doctors.
• If you have a particular clinical question in mind, check out the Signpost system — a free web-based resource provided by the Wessex Institute for Health Research and Development (http://www.signpoststeer.org). It helps you structure your question in a way that makes searching easier, and then provides links to literature sources relevant to your question.
• Did you know that the BMA offers a CD-ROM database of health-related newspaper cuttings? If you need infor-

mation about something that was in the press, call the BMA on 020-7387 4499.
• Learn how to do critical appraisal on what you read so that you can evaluate studies yourself, rather than relying on the authors' conclusions. It is little known that most published studies, even in leading medical journals, do not have reliable results because the study methodology was not rigorous enough. Critical appraisal is a simple process that enables you to be much more discriminating in what you read (see below in Evidence-based medicine).

Evidence-based medicine

Evidence-based medicine is being introduced into teaching hospitals around the country as this book goes to print. Basically, evidence-based medicine involves using research findings to give clinicians much more statistical power in interpreting everyday clinical data, rather than relying on anecdotal evidence. It may not sound like much, but most people find that evidence-based medicine markedly improves the way they practise medicine.

The idea of evidence-based medicine is not new. People have been using 'the literature' for years to improve clinical decision-making. However, the advent of big electronic databases such as MEDLINE, the CL and *Clinical Evidence* (see above) now mean that doctors can rapidly search and evaluate the literature on a regular and systematic basis, especially if these databases are installed on ward and library computers.

Not only do people who practise evidence-based medicine find that they become more aware — and critical — of research findings, but they quickly

* Milne R., Chambers L. (1993) Assessing the scientific quality of review articles. *Journal of Epidemiology and Community Health* **47**, 169–170.

become adept at solving difficult problems and find they can engage better in medical debates. Evidence-based medicine can be practised by teams or by individuals. Find out about it and try it out!

What does evidence-based medicine involve?

Evidence-based medicine involves carrying out three key steps:

1 Ask a clear question about the problem you are trying to solve (e.g. should I anticoagulate an elderly woman with asymptomatic atrial fibrillation?).

2 Search the literature for good quality evidence using a structured, hierarchical search that gives you the most statistically powerful research first. Stop when you have enough information to answer your question. Search first for systematic reviews, second for randomized controlled trials, and lastly for other types of studies. To do this efficiently you need access to an electronic database such as the CL and MEDLINE. See your hospital librarian or tap into them through the BMA or server if you have a computer and modem.

3 Critically appraise (or evaluate) the evidence you have found to see whether or not its findings are reliable and relevant to your situation. To do this you need a list of questions, which help you to assess the methodology of the research. These questions are available in: Oxman A.D., Sackett D.L., Guyatt G.H. Users Guides to the Literature I–III, *Journal of the American Medical Association* (1993) **207**, 2093; (1994) **271**, 59; (1994) **271**, 389.

These simple guides take you through the steps of critical appraisal for different kinds of research evidence.

To get to grips with evidence-based practice and critical appraisal, a user-friendly, inexpensive reference manual is: Sackett D.L., Haynes R.B., Guyatt G.H., Tugwell P. (1991) *Clinical Epidemiology. A Basic Science for Clinical Medicine*. 2nd edn. Little, Brown and Company, Toronto. It teaches you how to critically appraise different kinds of evidence including reviews, economic analyses and research about quality of care, therapy, diagnosis, screening, prognosis and disease causation.

Professionalism

No-one teaches you how to be a professional. Don't worry if the transition from student to doctor is full of bumps and jolts—it certainly was for us! There isn't much mystery to being 'professional'; it's mostly about communicating well, building relationships and being responsible for what you say and do. However, this is no small thing to accomplish.

Communication

For an enjoyable house job, good communication is essential. As a House Officer, you will make about 30 phone calls for every patient you admit. You may interview up to 5000 people during the year. You will write volumes of notes that others will rely on and that might one day be used as evidence in court. You will physically touch hundreds of people.

Unfortunately, many medical schools do not teach communication or relationship skills: you are supposed to pick them up from your seniors. As you have probably already observed, many seniors are singularly lacking in personal and communication skills. It pays to develop your own skills; they will save you bleeps, headaches, time, and law suits. Over 90% of UK medical defence cases result from poor communication rather than from negligence *per se*. Most so-called ward 'personality clashes' can be solved by effective and imaginative communication.

1 It is really important *and* difficult to write legibly at 3 am. Write for others as you would have things written for you. A fountain pen can force you to write legibly.

2 Write your name and bleep number on ward boards. This is very helpful for the nursing staff if you are on call (e.g. 14 May cover: Jo Bloggs' bleep 1413).

3 Let people know if you are very distressed about something. Try not to transform grief or fatigue into defensive behaviour, such as silence or arrogance. People are usually pretty good at helping you out if they know what's up.

4 ESP is not a reliable form of communication; short notes and phone calls work much better.

5 We have all been yelled at unreasonably by colleagues at some time. Try not to take it to heart or to say something you will later regret. There are a lot of disillusioned and depressed folk out there, just bristling for a fight. If they do have a legitimate point underlying their intemperance, learn the lesson and move on. That said, if you experience sustained and unprofessional bullying from another member of staff (which does happen in hospitals), you should seek to stop it, either by standing up to the person concerned (easier said than done) or by taking the problem to a trusted senior or

manager. The BMA helpline can assist with such things, too, for example by helping to identify who to take the case to next.

6 Most junior doctors lose their heads from time to time. Don't be afraid to say you're sorry. People usually respect apologies.

7 If conflicts arise, some useful tips include:*
- Ask yourself, are you sure you're right?
- Does it matter?
- Try turning difficult questions back to the patient. For example, you can ask them: 'What makes you ask that question?'†
- Try to appear calm, despite what you may feel inside.

8 There are many resources to help people understand choices about treatments more thoroughly, such as videos, pamphlets and on-line information. Contact a lecturer nurse, librarian or district health authority to find out if any are readily available.

9 Use an interpreter if necessary. Interpreters can usually be contacted through the switch board or the casualty nursing staff.

Consultants and senior registrars

- Each consultant will have about five things **they want to know** about each

---

* Hope R.A. *et al.* (1994). *Oxford Practice Skills Project: sample teaching materials.* Oxford Medical School, Oxford.
† Macguire P., Faulkner A. (1988) Communicate with cancer patients: Handling bad news and difficult questions. *British Medical Journal* **297**, 970–974.

patient (sometimes for no apparent reason). Find these out early and supply them tirelessly, no matter what they are. Your predecessor is usually a good source of this kind of information.

• NEVER say you've done something when you haven't.

• Impress your seniors by being straightforward and by knowing your patients well. This matters much more in your house job than having read the latest *NEJM*.

GPs

You will talk and write to many GPs; some you will get to know quite well. The following are some recommendations from a number of GPs, including Joe Rosenthal, a GP who also teaches at the Royal Free Hospital in London:

1 Phone requests for admission:
  • Have paper and pen ready.
  • Be polite.
  • Listen first.
  • Take down: Name
                 Age
                 Problem
                 Hospital number
                 GP name and
                   number
                 Expected time of
                   admission.

• Ask for a list of the patient's medications, particularly if the patient may be confused.

• Inform casualty.

2 Phone the GP on discharge if the patient:
  • Self-discharges.
  • Is in an unstable condition.
  • Has poor home circumstances.
  • Dies.
  • Needs an early visit.

3 Discharge letter. Complete before the patient leaves! Include:
  • Patient details.
  • Name of consultant.
  • Name of ward.
  • Diagnosis and important negative findings.
  • Treatment given.
  • Treatment on discharge.
  • Follow-up arrangements.
  • What the patient has been told.
  • Your name and bleep number.

4 Think about the resources the GP has in his or her surgery. Try to avoid things like 'repeat CXR in one month' on the discharge form. The GP is not an out-patient service. If there are loose ends requiring tests in future, set up a clinic appointment.

Nurses

It is pretty crucial to get on with nurses, who are fantastic allies. They know most of what you need to know as an House Officer and are usually keen and willing to teach you. Nurses are trained in a range of things that doctors aren't and vice versa, so the teams are complementary—use this to your advantage! Here are some hints for starters:

• Always introduce yourself to nurses and other staff when you're new on a ward.

• Always tidy up after yourself. Especially tidy up your own sharps. Most needlestick injuries arise from sharps someone else left hidden.

• Tidy up your trolley after any procedure. Find out in the first couple of weeks how to make up your own trolley and how to pack it away.

• Don't expect nurses to do things they are not qualified to do. Nurses may have

extended roles (such as IV drug administration) but they may not. Nurses can
be struck off much more easily than
doctors.

• Do unto nurses as they do to you.
Make them cups of tea or coffee or offer
to do an IV round if you're on the ward
without much to do. This helps to create
an easy, generous atmosphere on the
ward, which makes coming to work
much more fun.

• To avoid heaps of bleeps, ask nurses to
write down tasks and have one nurse
bleep you with the list every couple of
hours or so. Tell them you will return to
do a round at a specific time.

• If you foresee problems with a patient
overnight, discuss these with the nurses.
Arrange 'bleep thresholds' for foresee-
able problems. Instructions such as 'call
me if his systolic falls below 100' may
seem superfluous, but they suggest
that you are on top of the problem and
indicate your willingness to respond
promptly. This reduces the frequency of
those 'just thought you might like to
know...' bleeps.

• If multiple bleeps are a real problem,
consider arranging a meeting with the
medical or surgical manager and nursing
staff to work out a better system. This is
the sort of thing hospital managers are
employed for. Talk to your senior if he or
she is supportive.

• If you have a plan in your head for
a patient, or you foresee a problem a
patient might have (e.g. a delayed discharge date), let the nursing, social work
and occupational therapy staff know so
they can help you with it, rather than
having to nag you for information.

• Write instructions to nurses in the
medical notes.

• Save time: get to know how team

nursing works on your ward. Basically,
team nursing means that nurses work in
independent, often colour-coded teams,
each of which looks after a certain
number of patients. Do not try to elicit
information about a 'red' patient from a
'green' nurse (see below under Team
nursing).

• Nurses often work in three 8-hour
shifts. Their rota is usually kept in the
nurses' office. It is often helpful to know
when a particular nurse will be available.

• Try not to interrupt nurses when they
are meeting for the shift 'report', on han-
dover, or on their breaks.

Helpful things to know about nurses

• Nursing grades (varies between
hospitals):

   Student nurse: attends university for
   3–4 years (4 years if a degree course).

   Staff nurse: graded D–F (A–C are
   auxiliary nurses).

   Sisters: graded F–H (usually).

   Nurse managers: graded H–J.

   Lecturer practitioner: senior specialist
   nurse who teaches and advises more
   inexperienced staff. Nurse practitioners (extensively used in North
   America) are gradually increasing in
   number but are still relatively thin on
   the ground in the UK.

• Nursing jargon:

   Bank nurse is a nurse hired temporari-
   ly from a 'bank' agency.

   Charge nurse is a male version of ward
   sister.

   Team nursing means that nurses
   work in colour-coded teams, each of
   which independently cares for different groups of patients. It means
   that nurses get to know their patients
   better. It also means that nurses may

not know much about patients who aren't assigned to their team. If you want to know about a 'blue' patient, ask a 'blue-team' nurse.

To 'special' is to provide intensive nursing for a seriously ill patient.

Ward sister is the female version of charge nurse who may have overall responsibility for the patients.

Back/Late shift is the shift from approximately 2 pm to 9 pm.

Early shift is the shift from approximately 7 am to 2 pm.

• Things nurses hate most:

Doctors treating them like second class citizens.

Doctors not answering bleeps reasonably quickly (so they have to wait by the phone for ages).

Doctors leaving sharps (and other rubbish) around.

Doctors not explaining things well to patients and not informing the nurse what they found out from the patient.

Patients (see also p. 90, Breaking bad news)

• Listen to patients, even if you think their worries are trivial. Remember that you don't have to solve all their problems. Just listening can be a huge help.

• If you do not have time to listen to a patient properly, either organize for someone else to listen (such as their nurse) or tell the patient that you will sit down with them later. Preferably give the patient a time and stick to it.

• If you cannot make it back to talk to a patient, phone their nurse to tell the patient so they are not left waiting.

• Avoid medical jargon when talking to patients (for example, 'blockage' not 'stenosis').

• Give people information in bite-size chunks that they can manage. This is especially important for people who are anxious or when you are relaying scary information.

• Use conceptually clear diagrams wherever possible to explain yourself, as shown in Appendix B (remember that anatomically correct diagrams may be more confusing than conceptually clear ones).

• Be straightforward with patients. Answer questions honestly, even if it means saying that you don't know.

• Do not be pushed into committing yourself to a diagnosis or prognosis if you do not have good evidence for it.

Patients' families

Patients' families suffer terribly from lack of information from hospital staff. You can greatly alleviate this with minimal effort and you will be showered with gratitude. If possible, take the patient's nurse with you to ensure continuity of care. There are two main problems you can help with: patient discharge and informing families about their relative.

Information about patient discharge

Making arrangements for home care can be a major ordeal, particularly for families where everyone works. You should start thinking about the logistics from the moment the patient is admitted. You can make a big difference if you or the nurse can let the family know as soon as possible:

1 When (and if) the patient can go home; if possible, morning or afternoon. It may be possible for your patient to leave at a time that is convenient for family routines.

2 Special instructions that the patient will need to follow at home and when they should go and see their GP.
3 Drugs that will be needed and when in the near future.
4 Who they can contact if something goes wrong.
5 What you have asked the GP to arrange in the near future.

Hints

• Find out the discharge procedure from nurses.
• Be aware of hospital visiting hours so that you can tell families when patients are admitted.
• Liaise with nurses, social workers and occupational therapists, as they often have important information for patients and their families on discharge.
• Remember that many people will not challenge a doctor and may endure a lot of hassle to do what you say, even when it makes no difference to the ward. If families are looking bothered, ask them what's wrong. You may be able to help with little effort.
• Imagine the patient was your relative and you had to look after them—what would you need to know?
• Ask family members if they have any questions.

Information about what's wrong with the patient (see p. 90, Breaking bad news)

Your main duty is to care for the patient, not their family; you should get the patient's permission before divulging information to any family member. Taking time in a non-stressful environment to explain things to family members can be invaluable. Families remember how doctors explained things to them. Key features that we find make a difference include:
• Take the family to a private room. This enables people to remember information and ask questions.
• Try to get rid of your bleep. Hand it to a colleague.
• Have all investigations and findings to hand. Be ready to answer lots of questions and be ready to admit uncertainty.
• Write in the notes what you have told the family and tell the nursing staff.
• Have tissues and cups of tea handy if possible.
• If possible, collect all family members for one chat. Otherwise they turn up at all sorts of times and you have to repeat yourself.
• If news is very bad or unexpected, it may be courteous to ask your senior to see the family first.

Confidentiality

Breaches of confidentiality may be both unlawful and amount to professional misconduct, and you may be called upon to justify any such breach. Keeping confidentiality is not always as easy as it sounds—you may need to discuss patient histories with many people, both within the hospital and the community. The following guidelines should help you to keep legal confidentiality:
• Refer to patients by name as little as possible.
• Do not discuss confidential information with people over the phone unless you are certain of their identity and that they are authorized to receive the information.
• Never discuss patients in public

places, such as lifts and hospital canteens.

• *Never* discuss anything with the press if approached. Refer immediately to your consultant or the hospital manager.

• Refer police officers to your senior.

• Take care when discussing patients over the phone. Transfer ward calls to the doctors' office wherever possible. It is easy to find yourself shouting above the noise of a ward only to find that the entire ward can hear you.

• Remember that curtains are not sound proof. If you have confidential or delicate information to convey or obtain, consider taking the patient to a side room.

• Do not talk about patients so that they may be identified outside of immediately relevant hospital settings. For example, don't tell your dinner guests stories about patients that they may recognize, even if you don't name them. It is better to avoid this kind of thing altogether, however entertaining it may be.

• The MDU and MPS both have 24-hour advice lines if you are a member.

Exceptions to keeping confidentiality

There are common-sense exceptions to confidentiality, such as when you have good reason to believe that the patient is likely to cause death or serious harm to him- or herself or others. Sometimes it may not be clear cut as to whether you should or shouldn't respect confidentiality. For example, if a patient admits a crime to you, should you tell anyone about it? Whichever is the case:

• Always ask your consultant for advice.

• Document your decision and other relevant information in the notes to cover yourself in the event of a court case, or complaint. Your medical defence insurer can advise you if you are in any doubt.

Consent (see p. 189)

Chapter 6: **Cardiac arrests and crash calls**

You will almost certainly be a junior member of the hospital crash team. If you are first on the scene, the absolute priority is to ensure adequate ventilation and perfusion—basic life support. It is one occasion when a well-learnt plan of action is essential.

You do not have time to 'make a diagnosis'. Stay calm and then:

1 Make sure the airway is clear and secured and that someone (preferably two people working in rotations) is doing adequate CPR. Help if necessary. Basic life support guidelines are available at www.resus.org.uk/pages/bls.htm.

2 Secure IV access if basic life support is already being provided and there is a 'spare pair of hands' but do not waste time if you are struggling to put in an IV line. Get help fast and do point 3 in the meanwhile.

3 Get an ECG trace. If there is no chest lead monitor, this is quickly done by placing the defibrillator paddles over the chest.

Decide on a course of action according to the algorithm in Fig. 6.1; based on the new Advanced Life Support (ALS) guidelines (Resuscitation Council (UK) 2000). We strongly recommend you read the guidelines in full (available at www.resus.org.uk/pages/als.htm or from the ALS course coordinator in your hospital).

Hints

1 Find out on day one of your job how the defibrillator works and learn the layout of your hospital's arrest trolley. Enrol yourself on an advanced life support (ALS) course as soon as possible.

2 Note the time of the crash call so you can keep track of how long the resuscitation has been in progress.

3 Go to bed dressed in surgical scrubs if you are carrying the crash bleep. Time does matter and should not be wasted getting 'properly' dressed.

4 It is useful to know the patient's medical background although this is not a priority. Especially look for risk factors of:

- Exsanguinating bleed (e.g. oesophageal varices, recent surgery, bleeding disorder).
- Pneumothorax (e.g. recent central line placement, surgical procedures).
- Pericardial tamponade (e.g. recent chest trauma, recent MI).
- Pulmonary embolus (e.g. recent DVT, major pelvic surgery).
- MI (e.g. history of IHD).
- Electrolyte imbalance, especially K^+ levels (e.g. anuric patient after major surgery, patient with severe renal impairment).
- Drug overdose.

5 Cardiac arrest is traumatic for other patients on the ward. Use professional language and stay calm.

6 After an unsuccessful call, be sensitive

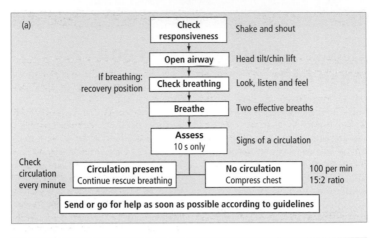

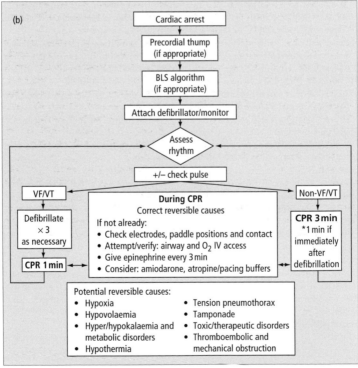

Fig. 6.1 Protocol for (a) basic and (b) advanced adult life support. Reproduced with permission from The Resuscitation Council (UK).

to the fact that nurses and other doctors may have a close relationship with the patient.

7 It is always worth checking that the patient is not 'not for resus in the event of cardiac arrest'. This should always be written clearly in the notes (see 'DNR orders' below). When in doubt, your duty is to attempt to save the patient's life.

'Do not resuscitate' orders

This is a complex area and a frequent cause of complaint and litigation. It is one of the most common reasons for the GMC to take doctors to task. Make sure you read the joint statement from the BMA and the Resuscitation Council (available at www.resus.org.uk/pages/dnr3.htm or from the BMA medical ethics department—tel. 0207 383 6286, email ethics@bma.org.uk). The key points are as follows:

1 The decision not to resuscitate should only be considered when the likelihood of success is very small.

2 Your consultant is responsible for resuscitation status. Do not change a patient's resuscitation status (in either direction) without discussing the case with your senior. Always document that

you have done so in the notes and state the rationale for the decision. Document the decision clearly—don't use codes like 'not for 222'

3 Good communication is essential. All decisions should be discussed with the entire medical team, the nursing staff, the patient (providing he or she is mentally competent) and the family.

4 The decision should take into account the views of the family, close friends, and staff. However, the bottom line is that only a competent patient may decide their status. If the patient is mentally incompetent or defers to the medical team, the consultant is then responsible for the decision.

5 If the patient has given an advance directive ('living will') while mentally competent, this must be followed, even if the patient is now mentally incompetent.

6 'Not for resus' does not preclude measures short of resuscitation (this may have to be explained to the family).

7 Resuscitation status should be reviewed in the light of changes to clinical condition.

8 In the event of an arrest where the status is unclear, resuscitation should be attempted.

9 If in doubt about these guidelines, ring your defence union (they have helplines for just such difficulties).

Chapter 7: **Common calls**

This section provides help with problems you are likely to get bleeped for. In particular, it helps you to exclude serious conditions and to initiate mainstay management.

How to use this section

Like a recipe book, this section lists basic protocols for common calls. We recommend the following:

• When first using the chapter, read the short blurb immediately beneath each call, which lists the most likely causes of each problem and things to watch out for. Differential diagnoses are listed in the way that makes them easiest to remember. Most of the time, this is in order of likelihood in the hospital setting.

• Feel free to scribble in the margins and make modifications to each 'recipe' in light of the clinical context and seniors' preferences. You probably will not need to carry out each step for every patient.

• To make this section easy to use in the middle of the night, we have kept abbreviations to a minimum. If in doubt, please refer to the abbreviations list (p. xiv). Drug abbreviations are as follows:

od	once in 24 hours
bd	twice in 24 hours
tds	three times in 24 hours
qds	four times in 24 hours
PO	orally

SC	subcutaneously
IM	intramuscularly
IV	intravenously
nocte	at night
mane	in the morning
stat	straight away
T., T.T.	one tablet, two tablets

Considerations for all ward calls

• Never hesitate to call your seniors. It is their job to back you up. However, like everyone else, seniors do not like to feel dumped on. Unless it is a dire emergency, make sure you have assessed the problem thoroughly and if possible make a provisional differential diagnosis and management plan.

• If you need help, always refer problems upwards (to seniors) not sideways (to other House Officers).

• Always examine patients in a good light even if it means switching on the main lights.

• Even in dire emergencies, act steadily and reassure the patient. If you need urgent senior help, stay with the patient and ask someone else to get hold of your senior.

• The key to managing simultaneous bleeps is to prioritize tasks according to urgency and location in the hospital.

• Keep emergency routines fresh in your mind throughout the year. Patients can deteriorate when you least expect it, such as on convalescent wards.

• Before going to bed, check that you know where to find: ophthalmoscope/otoscope; stethoscope; patella hammer; blood-taking equipment; catheter sets; blood gas machines; ECG machine; and blood fridges.

• While on call, wear respectable pyjamas such as theatre scrubs.

• If you are tired or woken from a deep sleep, try washing your face in cold water and mentally preparing yourself for the problem you are about to deal with. Consider differential diagnoses as you walk to the ward.

• After seeing patients, sit down with their notes and review their history to make sure you have not missed something, and document your findings.

• Whatever you are called for, don't forget to check the fluid and drug charts.

• When tired, try not to argue with nursing or medical colleagues. If you feel you are being bleeped unnecessarily, take the matter up when you are well rested.

• Do not be too hard on yourself if everything seems daunting. It is! Experience is the only way to develop good clinical judgement and familiarity with practical procedures.

Abdominal pain

Your priority is to exclude peritonism and obstruction. Common causes of non-acute abdominal pain, such as UTI, constipation and post-op pain, are not life threatening but may require treatment.

When answering your bleep, ask for:

• BP, pulse and T.
• Dipstick urine for protein and blood.
• Keep the patient NBM.

Differential diagnoses
Intestinal obstruction
• Constipation
• Adhesions
• Hernia, volvulus, tumour

Peritonism
• Inflammation or infection of any intra-abdominal organ: pancreatitis, cholecystitis, appendicitis, diverticulitis
• Perforated viscus
• Complications of pregnancy
• Ruptured ectopic pregnancy (a life-threatening emergency)
• Other gynaecological causes (ovarian torsion, etc.)
• Leaking abdominal aortic aneurysm (a life-threatening emergency)
• Intestinal infarction

Peptic ulceration/gastritis

Extra-peritoneal causes
• Urinary retention
• UTI
• Wound abscess
• Basal pneumonia
• Inferior MI (often with associated N&V and bradycardia)
• Retroperitoneal bleed or abscess
• DKA

On the ward

1 See the patient immediately. If flat, call for senior help and commence basic life support. See 'The moribund patient', p. 74.
2 If the patient is stable, take a more thorough history and examine the patient. Don't forget to consider:

• Medical history: alcohol, diabetes,

IBD, IHD, recent procedures, previous surgery, and shingles.

• Pain—localization and radiation, onset, character, relieving/aggravating factors, associated symptoms.

• LMP and gynae history (previous peritonitis, pelvic surgery, pelvic inflammatory disease, and previous ectopic pregnancy. Intrauterine devices predispose to tubal pregnancy)

• PR and FOB.

• Extra-abdominal causes.

• Exclude *peritonism*: localized or generalized peritonitis: fever, guarding, rebound tenderness, absent bowel sounds.

• Exclude *obstruction*: no flatus, no bowel motion, vomiting, cramping abdominal pain and abdominal distension. Check hernial orifices.

3 Investigations to consider:

• FBC and INR.

• C&E, urea, Ca, amylase and glucose.

• G&S.

• ABGs if acutely unwell, or if you suspect pancreatitis or intestinal ischaemia (both cause a metabolic acidosis).

• Radiology: erect CXR (free air under diaphragm, pneumonia), supine/erect AXR (check for air–fluid levels, intestinal distension, calcifications, air in biliary tree).

• ECG and cardiac enzymes to rule out MI.

• MSU for UTI (a common cause of abdominal pain in hospital) and urinary dipstick for blood or protein.

Hints

• Do not delay analgesia. Opiates do not mask the rigidity and rebound tenderness of peritonism.

• Involve the surgical team early if necessary.

• Gastritis and non-perforating peptic ulcers can cause severe epigastric pain but not true peritonism. The pain is usually relieved within minutes by antacids.

• Consider bowel infarction in patients who are acutely unwell with abdominal pain in the absence of peritonism.

• Free air under the diaphragm may persist for more than a week after abdominal surgery or laparoscopy.

Anaemia

You will usually be called by the lab for gross anaemia. In this case, your immediate concerns are to exclude bleeding and heart failure. Chronic anaemia should always be investigated before transfusion unless the patient is acutely compromised, since donor blood may mask the cause (see Table 7.1). By far the commonest cause of anaemia in the UK (other than menorrhagia) is occult GI blood loss.

On the ward

1 See the patient and assess the need for transfusion. Try to avoid transfusion until the diagnosis is clear, unless:

• Hb is dangerously low (<6 g/dl), although it is still usually possible to take samples for investigation prior to transfusion.

• The patient has symptoms (feeling faint, SOB at rest, tachycardia, angina, postural hypotension or has had serious acute blood loss).

Table 7.1 Differential diagnoses of anaemia.

Low MCV (<76 fl)	Normal MCV (76–96 fl)	High MCV (>96 fl)
Iron deficiency	Acute blood loss	B_{12} or folate deficiency
Bleeding (GI, vaginal)	Haemolysis	Liver disease
Nutritional	Chronic infection or	Alcoholism
Thalassaemia	inflammation	Marrow infiltration
Sideroblastic anaemia	Malignancy	Hypothyroidism
	Pregnancy	Reticulocytosis
	Renal failure	Acquired sideroblastic anaemia

Where possible, avoid transfusions in patients with:
• Haemoglobinopathies, especially thalassaemia. They can usually cope with low Hbs. Consult with your senior and haematologist.
• B_{12} deficiency, as it may precipitate heart failure.

2 Take a history and examine the patient. Do not forget to consider:
• Occult GI bleeding—dyspepsia, weight loss, change in bowel habit.
• Menorrhagia.
• Medication (NSAIDs, drugs causing haemolysis, marrow suppression).
• Recent procedures or operations.
• Jaundice, skin rashes, lymph nodes.
• Abdomen: splenomegaly, ascites.
• PR and FOB.
• CVS—signs of infective endocarditis, prosthetic valves.
• CNS—signs of peripheral neuropathy or dementia (B_{12} deficiency on alcoholism).

3 Investigations to consider:
• Repeat FBC and reticulocyte count.
• G&S or cross-match.
• Iron studies (iron, ferritin, total iron binding capacity, transferrin saturation), B_{12}, folate and blood film.
• C&E, urea, liver function tests.

• LDH as a useful marker of haemolysis.
• Other tests (e.g. bone marrow biopsy), according to the differential diagnoses.

Hints

• Patients with chronic anaemia are particularly susceptible to heart failure following transfusion. Check for existing heart conditions; discuss with your seniors first and transfuse them as slowly as possible.
• Iron-deficiency anaemia is not an end diagnosis—you need to investigate its cause. The commonest are occult GI blood loss due to peptic ulcer disease or colonic tumours; menorrhagia; poor diet; and pregnancy.
• Be alert to mild anaemia when checking routine blood results. Slight Hb deficits are easy to miss and can be an early sign of serious disease.
• Leukoerythroblastic anaemia means there are primitive red and white cells in the peripheral circulation. The patient may need a bone marrow biopsy and investigation for occult malignancy.
• Consider intra- and retroperitoneal bleeding in people with acute anaemia and no evidence of external haemor-

rhage. Look for bruising in the flanks or around the umbilicus.

Arrhythmia

While abnormalities in the heart rate and rhythm are relatively common and seldom life threatening, never be afraid to call the crash team *before* the patient arrests! You are not expected to diagnose and manage arrhythmias without senior advice.

When answering your bleep

Ask nursing staff for pulse, BP and T and to give O_2 if the patient is unwell.

Initial management for all arrhythmias

On the ward

1 See the patient. Check ABC. If flat, have someone call the crash team and commence CPR. Give 100% O_2.
2 If the patient is well and stable, take a brief history and examination. Do not to forget to consider:
  • Cardiac symptoms (chest pain, palpitations, breathlessness, nausea, syncope, swollen ankles) and heart conditions (IHD, MI, valvular heart disease, rheumatic fever).
  • Pulse rate and rhythm.
  • Circulatory status. Is the patient shut down? (low BP, cold peripheries, sweaty).
  • Signs of cardiac failure (raised JVP, peripheral oedema, basal inspiratory crackles, gallop rhythm—third and/or fourth heart sounds).

3 Do an ECG, and compare with previous ones.
4 Scan the patient's notes for details of current condition and treatment.
5 Document your findings and notify your senior.

Managing specific arrhythmias

Managing specific arrhythmias requires treatment of any underlying cause of cardiac decompensation, precise ECG diagnosis and correction of metabolic derangement. Use this section as a guide only. Local drug and consultant preference may markedly alter management. House Officers are not expected to diagnose or treat specific arrhythmias without senior advice.

Arrhythmias when the pulse is irregular with a NORMAL rate

Atrial fibrillation (normal rate)
Wandering atrial pacemaker
Ventricular ectopics
Variable AV block

On the ward

1 Severe symptoms are unusual. First do an ECG and then examine the patient. Atrial fibrillation and ectopics are common. Check the notes and find the most recent ECG for comparison. Is this a new problem?
2 In most cases, the arrhythmia is not significant. However, if the ECG reveals atrial fibrillation or multiple, frequent ectopics:
  • Examine the patient for heart failure (raised JVP, basal crackles,

swollen ankles) and mitral valve disease (murmurs, added sounds).
• Consider thyroid disease.
3 Investigations to consider:
• C&E, FBC, ESR, serial cardiac enzymes.
• Serial ECGs (AF is common post-MI).
• Consider T_4, TSH, digoxin levels and an ECHO.
Discuss further management with your senior.

Hints

• A normal peripheral pulse may coexist with a fast central heart rate. Measure and document both.
• AF is associated with MI, IHD, mitral valve disease, thyroid disease, hypertension, pericarditis and other causes of a dilated atrium. Rarely, it is associated with atrial myxoma, infiltration, endocarditis and rheumatic fever. It is common following cardiac surgery, when it is usually temporary.

Bradyarrhythmias (arrhythmias with a SLOW rate)

Sinus bradycardia
Sudden stress, severe pain, post-systemic infection
Inferior MI
AV heart block
  Second-degree heart block: intermittent block with or without an elongated P–R interval
  Third-degree heart block: complete heart block (no relationship between P waves and the QRS complex)
Drugs: amiodarone, beta-blockers, calcium channel blockers, digoxin
Faulty sinus node: sick sinus syndrome, infiltration
Hypothyroidism and hypothermia
Raised ICP
Jaundice

On the ward

1 See the patient and assess ABC. Bradycardic arrhythmias can be serious. *If flat*, call the crash team and start CPR if necessary. Give 100% O_2.
2 If the patient is stable but symptomatic, inform your senior and:
• Consider urgent ECG and C&E.
• Review all 'suspect' drugs (see above).
• If symptomatic with sinus bradycardia or AV block, give atropine 0.6 mg IV (up to 3 mg in 24 hours). If bradycardia continues, get help. Consider starting an isoprenaline infusion 1–3 µg/minute as a bridging measure while the patient waits for pacing.
• Consider urgent digoxin levels.
3 If the patient is asymptomatic, do an ECG and discuss further management with your senior.

Hints

• A fourth heart sound with bradycardia is common following inferior MI.
• A history of recent collapse requires urgent assessment even if the patient is currently asymptomatic.

Tachyarrhythmias (arrhythmias with a FAST rate)

Sinus tachycardia
Note that sinus tachycardia will have a regular rhythm
• Hypermetabolic states, e.g. fever, anxiety, hyperthyroidism
• Drugs: digoxin, nitrates, nicotine, sympathomimetics, theophylline
• Shock, sepsis or hypovolaemia of any cause
• Heart failure

Supraventricular tachycardia
• Atrial fibrillation with fast ventricular response (fast AF) (rhythm will be irregular)
• Atrial flutter (has regular rhythm; often 300 atrial beats per minute, with a ventricular response at 150 bpm, i.e. 1 : 2 conduction)
• Atrial tachycardia (has regular rhythm)
• WPW syndrome (rhythm is regular unless AF supervenes)
• Nodal (junctional) (rhythm is regular)

Ventricular tachycardia

On the ward

1 See the patient. Assess ABC. If flat, call the crash team, request an urgent ECG and start CPR if necessary. Give 100% O_2.
2 If the patient is stable, do an urgent ECG and consider a cardiac monitor. On the basis of the ECG, decide whether the patient has sinus tachycardia (normal wave form) or an arrhythmia.

• If the ECG reveals a sinus tachycardia, treat the underlying condition.
• If the ECG reveals an arrhythmia, you need to differentiate between SVT and VT, which can be difficult (see p. 45). Seek senior advice if you are unsure.

SVTs

• If the patient has SVT *and* hypotension, get help fast. The patient may require 50–100 J of *synchronized* DC cardioversion. Discuss transfer to CCU.
• The commonest cause of SVT without hypotension is atrial fibrillation (AF) (irregularly irregular pulse and no P waves on ECG). Common causes of fast AF in the hospital setting include MI, pulmonary embolus and pneumonia. First-line treatment is digoxin or cardioversion if the AF is of acute onset. Digoxin controls the ventricular rate, but does not cure the underlying fibrillation (see Drugs, p. 106, for initiating digoxin therapy).
• If the patient has SVT that is not AF, they may need immediate treatment, but discuss with your senior first. Most SVTs respond to IV adenosine. Ensure that the patient is on a cardiac monitor and that a resus trolley is close to hand. Inject 3 mg adenosine rapidly into a large peripheral or central vein. If there is no response after 1–2 minutes, give 6 mg, and then a further 12 mg if necessary. Expect facial flushing, transient breathlessness and nausea. Warn the patient that they may experience transient chest pain when you inject the adenosine.

VTs

• Treat pulseless VT in the same way

that you would VF (see advanced life support guideline, p. 36).

• Sustained VT usually precipitates shock unless treated with DC cardioversion (100–200 J), so seek urgent senior help. Note that a broad complex tachycardia may be SVT with bundle branch block but should be treated as VT until proved otherwise.

• Investigations to consider:

C&E, Ca, Mg, cardiac enzymes if recent onset, FBC if acutely unwell. Consider T$_4$ and TSH.

Drug levels as appropriate: digoxin, theophylline and anti-arrhythmics.

ABGs and CXR if acutely unwell.

Whether the patient has a VT or SVT, you need to identify and treat the underlying cause, in addition to treating the arrhythmia.

Hints

• In discriminating between SVT and VT:

SVTs have narrow complexes (<140 ms) and are not necessarily associated with serious underlying heart disease.

VTs have broad complexes (>140 ms) and always indicates serious underlying heart disease.

• Carotid sinus massage can cause sinus arrest, especially in the elderly, or if the patient has had a recent MI or is digitalized. Use only if urgent action is required.

• Atrial tachycardia with heart block is commonly associated with digoxin toxicity.

• In discriminating VT and SVT with bundle branch block (both of which cause a wide complex tachycardia):

A history of IHD strongly suggests VT.

QRS morphology looks similar in all the leads in VT, but different in SVT with BBB.

QRS and atrial activity are dissociated in VT, but associated in SVT with BBB (this may be difficult to see because of rate).

An irregular rate suggests fast AF with BBB.

If there are any narrow complex beats among the broad complex beats, it is VT (the narrow complexes represent the occasional normally conducted supraventricular beat—telling you that there is no BBB).

• If the patient is compromised and you are not sure, treat as VT while waiting for a second opinion.

Calcium

Most labs report *total* serum Ca, of which about half is bound to albumin. If the albumin levels are low the lab result will underestimate total Ca. To correct roughly for hypoalbuminaemia, add *0.02 × the albumin deficit* to the laboratory result, or ask for an ionized Ca level which need not be adjusted for albumin (a special tube is required). Albumin deficit is defined as *40 – measured albumin level*.

Hypercalcaemia

On the wards, this is often spurious and often an incidental finding. However, true hypercalcaemia may need to be corrected. Rarely, it requires urgent treatment.

Differential diagnoses
• Spurious: tourniquet left on too long or blood taken from the drip arm
• Hyperparathyroidism (primary and tertiary)
• Malignancy—bony metastases, myeloma, paraneoplastic syndrome
• Drugs—thiazide diuretics, excessive ingestion of Ca-containing antacids, excessive vitamin D intake
• Rarer causes: granulomatous diseases (e.g. sarcoid, TB), endocrinopathies

On the ward

1 See the patient. Check that the result reflects true hypercalcaemia. In hospital, hypercalcaemia is usually an incidental finding and is frequently 'spurious', due to dehydration, venous stasis, taking blood from an infusion arm or abnormal albumin (see above). However, a corrected Ca of above 3.5 mmol/l usually requires treatment.

2 Exclude acute symptoms which require urgent treatment (anorexia, vomiting, abdominal pain, impaired mental state, dehydration). If acutely symptomatic:
• Seek senior advice.
• Consider: saline diuresis: 3–6 l normal saline/24 hours IV and furosemide (frusemide) 40–120 mg 2–4-hourly according to response. A CVP and urinary catheter is useful to monitor fluid balance (a catheter is also kinder if the patient has difficulty getting to the loo).
• Avoid phosphates until Ca levels are normal or risk deposition of Ca phosphate ('metastatic Ca/Pi deposition').
• Consider hydrocortisone (especially useful in malignancy, sarcoid and vitamin D intoxication), calcitonin or mithramycin therapy.

3 If the patient has true hypercalcaemia but is not acutely unwell:
• If dehydrated, request that the patient drink enough fluid to maintain a urine output of >2–3 l/day. If very dehydrated or unable to drink, consider IV fluids.
• Investigate the cause of hypercalcaemia, exclude renal impairment and correct abnormal K and Mg levels (see investigations below).
• Mobilize as soon as possible.

4 Investigations to consider:
• C&E, ESR, phosphate, alk phos, Mg.
• ECG. Review CXR.
• Consider plasma Igs, serum and urine electrophoresis, urinary Bence-Jones protein, skeletal survey, bone marrow biopsy (myeloma investigations) and PTH levels.

Hypocalcaemia

Like hypercalcaemia, hypocalcaemia can be spurious and may be caused by acute hyperventilation. Hypocalcaemia is rarely an emergency, unless Ca is <1.5 mmol/l (risking laryngo-spasm).

Differential diagnoses
• Spurious (low albumin, blood taken from drip arm)
• Acute hyperventilation
• Major systemic illness, especially pancreatitis
• Hypoparathyroidism—thyroid surgery or neck irradiation

continued

- On TPN without adequate Ca
- Vitamin D deficiency—malabsorption, renal disease, phenytoin or phenobarbitone
- Excessive ingestion of phosphate

On the ward

1 Assess the severity of the patient's condition. Check that the result is not spurious. Look for peripheral or oral paraesthesia, carpopedal spasm, Chvostek's sign (tapping over the facial nerve induces facial twitch), confusion and tetany.

2 If hypocalcaemia is symptomatic or Ca <1.5 mmol/l, seek immediate senior advice and institute treatment to prevent laryngospasm. Give 10% Ca gluconate 10–20 ml in 50–100 ml 5% dextrose over 5 minutes (not faster), followed by 1–2 mg/kg/h IV for 6–12 hours according to response. Correct the Mg deficiency and measure the phosphate level. If the phosphate is high, discuss with senior. The patient may need phosphate binders and slow correction of Ca, as too rapid correction can result in metastatic deposition of Ca phosphate.

3 Asymptomatic hypocalcaemia (Ca >1.75 mmol/l) does not require immediate treatment. Give oral supplements (2–4 g daily in divided doses) that contain cholecalciferol (most do—see the *BNF*).

4 Investigations to consider:
  - U&E, Mg, phosphate.
  - Others according to the differential diagnosis.

Hint

To avoid hypocalcaemia in patients on TPN, check Mg and Ca measurements at least weekly, and more frequently if acutely unwell.

Chest pain

Chest pain always requires urgent attention. While angina, oesophagitis and oesophageal spasm are the commonest causes of chest pain, never forget pulmonary embolus in the hospital setting.

When answering your bleep

Ask the ward staff to:
- Find an ECG machine.
- Repeat the vital signs.
- If the patient has a history of IHD, prescribe sub-lingual GTN 5 mg over the phone and start 40% O_2.

Differential diagnoses
Heart
- Angina (IHD, LVH/HOCM)
- Acute MI
- Pericarditis or myocarditis, including post-MI Dressler's syndrome

Lung/pleura
- Pulmonary embolus
- Pneumothorax
- Pleurisy/pneumonia

Aorta
- Dissection
- Aneurysm

GIT
- Oesophageal spasm
- Oesophagitis/gastritis
- Pancreatitis, cholecystitis, peptic ulcer

continued on p. 48

Other
- Shingles
- Costochondritis
- Rib or vertebral collapse

Sudden onset of central chest pain
- Exacerbation of IHD
- MI
- Oesophageal spasm
- PE or dissecting aneurysm
- Pneumothorax
- Rib fracture

On the ward

1 Assess the patient. If flat, get help (± crash team) and institute emergency treatment:
- 100% O_2.
- IV access.
- Urgent C&E, FBC, cardiac enzymes, ABGs.
- ECG (stat) and ECG monitor.
- Urgent mobile CXR.

2 If the patient is stable, take a more thorough history and examination. Do not forget:
- T, BP, pulse and circulation (well-perfused or cold and clammy?).
- The key to the diagnosis is the history. Specifically:
(a) Ask a lot about the pain itself. Have they had this pain before? Do they have known IHD or oesophagitis/oesophageal spasm? Does the pain feel anginal? Is it relieved by GTN? Relieving or precipitating factors (exercise, posture, food)? Pain lasting less than 30 seconds, stabbing or sharp in quality and highly localized is unlikely to be due to ischaemia.
(b) Any N&V (common with MI)? Recent falls or trauma?

- Listen for pleural and pericardial rubs (often missed).
- If there are odd chest noises, think of pneumothorax.

3 Investigations to consider:
- ECG ± CXR.
- IV access if you suspect an MI.
- Repeat ECG in 1–2 hours (there may be no ECG changes in an early MI).
- C&E and cardiac enzymes. Consider blood gases, FBC, clotting and G&S if embolus, anticoagulation or surgery is likely.

4 Discuss with your senior.

Hints

- Pain radiating to either arm, neck or jaw suggests a cardiac cause.
- Sub-lingual GTN provides immediate relief of angina and is a useful diagnostic aid. It also relieves oesophageal spasm, but over a few minutes.
- Oesophageal spasm or severe anxiety sometimes causes ischaemia-like changes on the ECG. Seek advice if unsure.

Confusion

Beware of unexpected confusion in patients. In particular, hypoxia is common, but easily missed in the elderly. Never assume disorientation or dementia without first excluding serious medical causes and ascertaining the patient's usual mental state.

When answering your bleep ask for:

- A ward blood glucose test (blood glucose stick).

- T, BP, pulse and urine dipstick.
- Pulse oximetry if available (p. 78).

Differential diagnoses

'DIM TOP' (Mike's South African acronym!)

D rugs (especially sedatives and analgesics)

I nfection (anywhere; commonly UTI and pneumonia)

M etabolic—hypoglycaemia, Na$^+$, K$^+$, Ca, liver or renal failure

T rauma (concussion, subdural haematoma)

T oxins (alcohol withdrawal, drugs, others)

O xygen deficit (hypoxia)—pneumonia, pulmonary oedema, PE, respiratory depression (opiates), anaemia

P ain and discomfort (any cause, including urinary/faecal retention)

P sychiatric/dementia

P erfusion abnormalities (CVA, TIA)

P ost-op confusion (hypoxia, urinary retention, infection, drugs, abnormal electrolytes, pain, blood loss, disorientation, alcohol withdrawal)

On the ward

1 Assess the patient's general condition and vital signs. If the patient is very agitated or violent, get help from nurses and porters. Consider sedation (5 mg diazepam i v is usually sufficient). Alternatively, use 5–10 mg haloperidol IM or PO or chlorpromazine 50–100 mg IM or PO (caution in cardiac patients). Have a resus trolley to hand. You may need to wait 10–20 minutes for the drug to take effect. In alcoholic patients consider clomethiazole instead (see p. 109).

2 If the patient is stable, take a history and examination. Don't forget to:
- Specifically exclude cardiac and respiratory distress. Breathe with the patient and consider a pulse oximeter reading or ABGs. Hypoxia is a surprisingly common cause of confusion that is easily missed.
- Perform a mini-mental test score. Is the patient truly confused or just disorientated, in pain or angry?
- Ask about recent falls, funny turns or previous strokes/TIAs. Is the patient in atrial fibrillation?
- Check possible infection sites (IV lines, UTI, chest, surgical wounds) and palpate for a full bladder or packed colon (urinary retention is a common cause of confusion). Look at the fundi for raised ICP (e.g. in subdural haematoma) and briefly assess the CNS for localizing signs.
- Check drug and fluid charts and review the medical background.

3 Ask the nursing staff or a relative about the patient's usual mental state. Is this a new occurrence?

4 Investigations to consider:
- C&E, glucose, FBC and ESR, ABGs.
- Blood cultures.
- Liver function tests (INR).
- Plasma Ca in patients with malignancy.
- ECG.
- CXR, CT head.

Hints

- Nurse the patient in a moderately lit room and minimize noise. Give repeated reassurance to the patient. A well-loved family member or a familiar nurse is invaluable.

• Consider nursing the patient on a mattress on the floor. Some hospitals have special 'soft walled' beds. Bed rails and 'hand ties' are regarded by most nursing staff as unnecessary and potentially dangerous.

• Secure NG tubes and IV lines with bandages. It is occasionally necessary to put mittens on the patient's hands.

• If you have excluded serious causes, consider short-term sedation with a benzodiazepine (diazepam 5–10 mg IV slowly, repeated after 4 hours if necessary). For shorter effect use lorazepam 1–2 mg (25–30 μg/kg) IV slowly, repeated after 6 hours if necessary. Use with caution in the elderly. Alternatives include:

Haloperidol 5–10 mg IM or PO
Chlorpromazine 50–100 mg IM or PO (caution in cardiac patients). (Both haloperidol and chlorpromazine are especially useful in the more acute setting. Have a resus trolley to hand. You may need to wait 10–20 minutes for the drug to take effect.)
In alcoholic patients consider clomethiazole instead (see p. 109).
Thioridazine 12.5–25 mg PO at night or 12 hourly is often used in geriatric units.

• You may not find any cause for the patient's confusion. Patients may simply be disorientated from a change in environment, but make sure you exclude serious medical causes before making this diagnosis. Clear, repeated explanation about where the patient is and why can be helpful, as is a small map showing where the toilets are and how to call for nursing assistance.

Constipation

Constipation is common in hospital due to hospital food, immobility, drugs and having to use a bedpan. It is more effective to treat the cause than to prescribe laxatives. Always be alert to obstruction and its causes (particularly tumours). Post-op ileus is common, usually resolves by itself and should never be treated with laxatives!

Differential diagnoses
Low roughage diet

Immobility

Drugs
• Aluminium or Ca-based drugs (e.g. antacids)
• Ca channel blockers (verapamil)
• Ferrous sulphate
• Opiates
• Tricyclic antidepressants
• Anticholinergics
• Slow K^+

Embarrassment at using a bedpan
GIT
• Pain (anal fissures, haemorrhoids, recent surgery)
• IBS
• Obstruction (acute and sub-acute) from any cause, especially tumours
• Ileus (pseudo-obstruction)

Metabolic
• Dehydration (especially in the elderly)
• Endocrine—hypothyroidism
• Hypercalcaemia, hypokalaemia

Neurological
• Spinal cord compression/lesions

On the ward

1 See the patient. Exclude:
- Intestinal obstruction (vomiting, abdominal pain or distension, high pitched bowel sounds). If present, consider tumour (see p. 39, Abdominal pain).
- IBD (which can cause constipation. Never prescribe laxatives in these patients without first consulting your senior).
- Pain or embarrassment which may inhibit straining. Have they had recent surgery?

2 Take a brief history and examination. Don't forget:
- To ask the patient how often they usually open their bowels. They may not have true constipation.
- PR (faecal impaction, anal fissure). Check for FOB.
- Drug and fluid charts.

3 Investigations are seldom necessary but consider:
- K^+, Ca, FBC.
- T_4 and TSH only if you suspect hypothyroidism.

4 Management. For simple constipation:
- Ensure adequate hydration and mobilize if possible.
- Bulk-forming agents: bran cereals or ispaghula husk (Fybogel or Metamucil).
- Stool softeners: docusate sodium (cheap) or lactulose (expensive).
- Stimulants: senna or bisacodyl. Glycerine suppositories if NBM. Co-danthrusate (danthron docusate) is effective but reserved for very elderly or terminally ill patients due to risk of danthron-induced GIT tumours.

- Enemas, e.g. phosphate enema 100 ml.

5 Consider prophylaxis for patients at risk of constipation (bedridden, e.g. post-op, CVA or patients on regular opiates):
- Stool softeners (docusate sodium 100 mg/day, or lactulose 10 ml/bd) and/or stimulants (senna 1–2 tablets daily) or enemas. Adjust doses in light of symptoms.

Diarrhoea

By far the commonest cause in hospital is drugs (antibiotics and laxatives) but infection should always be considered. Less common but important to consider is obstruction with overflow. In all cases, the patient may need to be rehydrated.

Differential diagnoses
- Anxiety and pain
- Drugs: laxatives, broad-spectrum antibiotics leading to *Clostridium difficile* infection (pseudo-membranous colitis), antacids containing Mg sulphate. Also cimetidine, colchicine, cytotoxic agents, digoxin, thiazide diuretics (see the *BNF*)
- Intestinal obstruction with overflow (neoplasm)
- Faecal impaction with overflow, especially in elderly patients
- Infection (immunocompromised? antibiotics? recent travel?)
- IBD, other causes of intra-abdominal inflammation, ischaemia, etc.
- Non-specific in association with other diseases

On the ward

1 Exclude severe dehydration (vital signs: BP lying and sitting, JVP, mucous membranes).

2 Directed history and examination:
- Risk for intra-abdominal sepsis (recent surgery, diverticular disease), IBD, immunocompromise (including HIV).
- N&V, blood or mucus PR.
- Peritonism or impaction.
- Drug chart for new drugs, laxatives, antibiotics.

3 If the patient is otherwise well and an infective cause is unlikely with no evidence of colitis or intra-abdominal mischief, send a stool sample for MC&S and prescribe an antidiarrhoeal agent, for example loperamide 4 mg initially, then 2 mg with each loose stool.

4 If the patient has systemic signs or is taking antibiotics:
- Take a fresh stool specimen for MC&S and *Clostridium difficile* toxin.
- Consider sigmoidoscopy and biopsy if the patient has bloody diarrhoea or the stool culture is negative.

5 Further investigations to consider:
- C&E; FBC to check WCC.
- Electron microscopy (EM) of stool specimen for viral infection (SSRVs).
- Inflammatory markers (CRP and ESR) especially if known IBD.
- Special cultures/stains for cryptosporidia, mycobacteria, etc., for immunocompromised patients.
- Plain abdominal X-ray (to look for colonic distension) if associated with pain or known IBD.

6 Irrespective of the cause you must ensure adequate hydration.

- Oral rehydration regime (see *BNF*—oral rehydration).
- IV fluids if severe or the patient cannot drink (see p. 62).

Hints

- Barrier nursing is advisable until infection is ruled out.
- Always wash your hands between patients.
- Be wary of diarrhoea in patients on steroids. Their abdomens may be 'silent' despite serious intra-abdominal mischief.

Electrocardiograms

Do not get too worried about interpreting ECGs during your house job. While the range of potential anomalies is bewildering at first, practice really does make perfect and House Officers are only expected to diagnose a handful of important conditions (see below). For a more complete guide consult Hampton's *ECG Made Easy* and *ECG in Practice* (see Bibliography, p. 2). Whatever the ECG diagnosis, remember to treat the patient, not the ECG!

> **Common ECG diagnoses**
> Atrial fibrillation (no P waves, rate can be fast or normal)
> Recent or past MI (see below)
> Third-degree heart block (no relationship between P waves and QRS complexes)
> Ventricular tachycardia
> Ventricular fibrillation

Basic ECG parameters to consider

- Rate: 60–90 bpm (lower in athletes)
- Rhythm: irregular or regular
- Axis: normal: −30 to +120° (some use 0 to +90)
- P waves: present/absent before each QRS complex?
- PR constant? Normal interval:120–200 ms (3–5 small squares)
- QRS up to 120 ms (3 small complexes: squares). Check height of the R waves Are Q waves present?
- ST isoelectric (i.e. on segment: baseline)?
- T waves: upright or inverted?

If the ECG is abnormal, consider each parameter systematically:

Abnormal rate and rhythm

Atrial tachycardia

- QRS rate >100/minute.
- Narrow QRS (<120 ms) (except in SVT with BBB or WPW syndrome).
- P wave abnormal (shape, size, upside down, swallowed by QRS, or with short PR interval).

Atrial fibrillation

- No P waves.
- Irregularly timed QRS complexes.

Atrial flutter

- Saw-tooth baseline of atrial depolarization.
- Regular QRS complexes.

AV nodal rhythm

- Narrow QRS complex.
- P waves hidden within the QRS complex or just preceding it (very short PR interval). P waves may be inverted.

Ventricular tachycardia

- Wide QRS (>120 ms), rate >150/minute.
- Abnormal T waves.
- P waves often absent or may have no relationship to QRS complexes.

Hint

If there is a rapid QRS rate without P waves, a wide QRS (>120 ms) indicates VT (unless there is pre-existing BBB) whereas a narrow QRS (<120 ms) indicates AV nodal tachycardia.

Calculating the axis

1 If the QRS is predominantly positive in I and II the axis is normal.
2 If not, find a lead in which the QRS complexes have equal positive and negative deflections. The axis lies 90° to that lead.
3 To determine the actual axis see Fig. 7.1.

P waves

1 Indicate atrial depolarization and are best seen in leads II and V1.

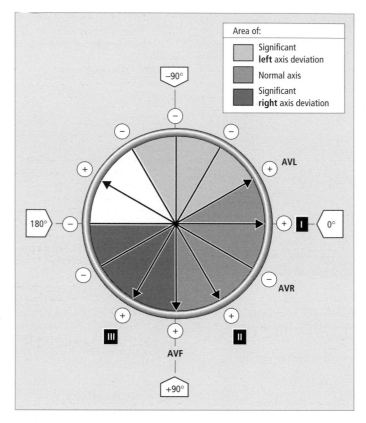

Fig. 7.1 Determining the axis for ECG examination.

2 Large left atrium (p. mitrale): bifid and wide (>110 ms), P wave in II, biphasic in V1.

3 Large right atrium (p. pulmonale): peaked P waves (>2.5 mm). Look at lead II.

4 No P waves: atrial fibrillation.

PR interval

Delay indicates abnormal AV conduction = HB.

1 First-degree HB: prolonged PR interval in each cycle but all P waves conducted.

2 Second-degree HB: some P waves are not followed by a QRS complex. May

find 2 (or 3) P waves before a QRS complex = 2:1 (or 3:1) block. P wave rate is normal. Progressive lengthening of the PR interval then non-conducted P wave is called the Wenckebach phenomenon.

3 Third-degree HB: no relationship between P waves and QRS complexes. Ventricular escape rhythm <50/minute. QRS usually wide.

4 A consistently short PR interval indicates conduction down accessory pathways (e.g. WPW). May be associated with 'slurred' upstroke of the QRS.

QRS complexes

Wide complexes (>120 ms) indicate abnormal ventricular depolarization, occurring in VT, ventricular extra-systoles, complete heart block or bundle branch block.

1 Ventricular extra-systoles: no P wave, early QRS and abnormally shaped QRS complex, abnormal T-wave. Next P wave is 'on time'. Isolated extra-systoles are a common normal finding (particularly in young, fit people). They should, however, become less frequent as a person exercises.

2 LBBB: RSR' 'W' pattern in V1, 'M' pattern in V6. Inverted T waves in I, a VL, V5–6 (remember the mnemonic 'WiLliaM'). The presence of LBBB may mask underlying infarction.

3 RBBB: RSR' 'M' pattern in V1, 'W' pattern in V6. Inverted T waves in V1–3, deep and wide S wave in V6 (remember the mnemonic 'MaRroW').

4 Ventricular strain/hypertrophy: inverted T waves and depressed ST segments in the appropriate chest leads (V1–3 for RV and V4–6 for LV).

5 RVH: R wave larger than S wave in V1 and no RBBB, deep S in V6. Sometimes right axis deviation. NB: a dominant R in V1 is seen in posterior infarction and RBBB.

6 LVH: R wave in V6 >25 mm in height or R wave in V6 + S wave in V1 >35 mm in height. Occasionally left axis deviation.

ST segment and T waves

1 Depressed ST segments: ischaemia, digoxin toxicity ('inverted tick' ST depression and inverted T waves in V5–6), posterior myocardial infarction.

2 Elevated ST segments (always serious): infarction, coronary artery spasm (variant angina), pericarditis/myocarditis (saddle-shaped ST segments in all leads), ventricular aneurysm, posterior ischaemia.

3 T wave inversion is often non-specific but in the context of chest pain points to critical ischaemia.

Important ECG abnormalities to recognize

Myocardial infarction

Sequence of changes (Table 7.2):
1 At first the ECG may be normal.

Table 7.2 Diagnosing infarction sites by ECG changes.

Site of infarction	Changes seen in leads
Anterior	V2–V5
Inferior	III and a VF
Lateral	I, a VL and V6
True posterior	Dominant R in V1 (exclude RV strain and RBBB)

2 Within 6 hours, tall T waves and raised ST segments are evident.

3 Within 24 hours, T waves invert and ST segments normalize.

4 After 24 hours, Q waves are evident and ST segments are normal.

NB: T wave inversion may or may not persist. Q waves persist.

Pulmonary embolism

There are often no ECG changes:

1 Sinus tachycardia.

2 Evidence of RV strain/hypertrophy (see above).

3 Right axis deviation.

4 RBBB.

5 Deep S in I, Q in V3, inverted T in V3 ('SI, Q3, T3').

Eye complaints

Except for the simplest problems, House Officers are not expected to diagnose or treat eye diseases. Do not be afraid to seek an ophthalmological opinion. Ophthalmologists are usually keen for referrals and can teach you a lot.

The acute red eye

Differential diagnoses
Conjunctivitis
Foreign body
Corneal ulceration/herpes keratitis
Acute glaucoma
Acute iritis

On the ward

1 Take a brief history and examination. Don't forget:

- Clinical background, especially diabetes and other systemic diseases.
- Visual acuity, discharge, corneal lustre.
- Pupils: shape, direct and consensual responses.
- Ophthalmoscopy to assess red reflex (normal in conjuctivitis and simple foreign body) and fundus.

2 Unless the cause is obvious, notify your senior and seek an urgent ophthalmological opinion.

- If the problem is unilateral, ask about previous history of shingles (look for periocular vesicles) or iritis (which often recurs in the fellow eye). Conjunctivitis or ulceration can also be unilateral.
- Exclude conjunctivitis: the eye usually feels itchy and tears. Vision, corneal lustre, pupillary responses and red-reflex are all normal. Purulent discharge suggests bacterial conjunctivitis. Look at the pattern of redness/injection. Intensity of injection around the periphery suggests conjunctival inflammation, whereas injection around the cornea suggests corneal or intra-ocular inflammation.
- Exclude acute glaucoma: the eye is red and painful, the pupil is hazy and fixed and the patient sees halos around lights. Seek urgent ophthalmological assistance.
- Exclude a foreign body: the eye usually tears. Foreign bodies are sometimes hidden under the inside of the upper lid. Invert the upper lid over a small spatula (cotton bud or orange stick). Bear in mind that the sensation of having a foreign body in the eye can also be caused by corneal ulcers and acute keratitis.

Sudden loss of vision in one or both eyes

This is always an emergency. Seek immediate ophthalmological advice.

> **Differential diagnoses**
> Acute glaucoma
> Central artery or vein occlusion
> Amaurosis fugax
> Optic neuritis
> Retinal detachment
> Severe hyperglycaemia
> Temporal arteritis

Floaters

Floaters are usually condensations of vitreous, but can be blood, bits of retina or inflammatory cells. They are normal with age, but if they have appeared recently or suddenly, seek an ophthalmological opinion.

Falls

While most falls in hospital are trivial, they are a common cause of fracture in the elderly. You need to sign an accident form when called to investigate a 'fall' (see p. 11).

When answering your bleep

• Consider asking for a ward glucose test.

> **Differential diagnoses**
> • Simple accident (slippery floor, disorientation, frailty, generalized weakness from illness)

• Poor vision (no glasses, cataracts)
• Drowsiness from drugs, especially sedatives and recent anaesthesia

Occasionally:
• Loss of consciousness: TIA, fit, vaso-vagal, postural hypotension, vasodilator and other drugs, cough/micturition syncope, arrhythmias/MI, PE, mitral/aortic stenosis, hypoglycaemia, anaemia
• Poor motor function/balance: generalized weakness from illness, Parkinson's disease, cerebellar disease, peripheral neuropathy, multiple sclerosis

On the ward

1 See the patient. Nurses are legally liable until the patient is seen by a doctor.
2 Ask the patient what happened and which part hurts the most. Don't forget:
   • T, pulse and BP, including postural drop.
   • Consciousness level (see Glasgow Coma Scale, p. 216) and mini-mental test score if appropriate.
   • Skin for bruising, bleeding, cuts and fractures.
   • Bone tenderness for fractures. Frail patients can sustain fractures with remarkably little fuss. Especially look for hip, wrist and scaphoid fractures. Examine the skull carefully if the patient has hit their head. If there are signs of head injury or drowsiness, consider a CT head (see p. 183).
   • Drug and fluid charts (sedatives, hypoglycaemic agents, vasodilators (especially ACE inhibitors), anti-arrhythmics).

3 Investigations to consider:
  • C&E, FBC (?raised WCC), glucose.
  • MSU.
  • ECG.
  • The patient may need cardiac investigations later (e.g. ECHO, 24-hour ECG).
4 Sign an accident form (ask the nurses for one). If the patient appears well, 'No apparent injuries on examination' is sufficient.
5 Write in the patient's notes. Include:
  • Time and date.
  • Brief history of accident.
  • Brief examination findings.
  • That you signed an accident form.
6 Ask the nurses to continue to do regular observations and to contact you if the patient's condition deteriorates. If the patient has hit their head, consider requesting neurological observations.
7 Think about what caused the fall. Make a plan with the nurses to prevent future accidents.

Hints

• Many falls are caused by patients being in an alien environment, particularly in elderly patients with poor righting reflexes. To prevent future falls, show patients the call button and remind them that they need to call the nurse for toilet assistance after anaesthetics or sedatives. If the bed needs to remain raised high off the floor, caution patients about the drop before stepping down onto slippery linoleum.
• Fractures or simple bruising in the elderly can lead to substantial blood loss. Never forget to check limbs for occult fractures.
• Sudden loss of consciousness is most commonly caused by fainting, postural

hypotension and arrhythmia. MIs rarely present with syncope alone.

Fever

In hospital, fever is most commonly due to infection, blood transfusions and drugs. When called at night, the major concern is to exclude bacterial infection.

Differential diagnosis

Infection, especially UTI, phlebitis, pneumonia. More common in diabetics

Drug-induced, especially antibiotics, allopurinol, ibuprofen. Common during blood transfusions

Thrombosis ± infarction: DVT, PE, MI, ischaemic bowel

Tumours

Alcohol withdrawal

Hyperthyroidism

Inflammatory and vasculitides, especially IBD, rheumatoid arthritis

Post-surgery

Think 4 Ws: Wind (i.e. respiratory), Wound (including lines), Water, Walking (DVT).

On the ward

1 See the patient. Check T, pulse and BP and check the charts. Fever above 40°C requires urgent action. If there is any chance of shock (tachycardia, hypotension with warm peripheries), ensure large-bore IV access and commence IV fluid resuscitation. Take blood cultures (at least two sets). Discuss IV broad-spectrum antibiotic cover with your senior.

2 Exclude immunosuppression and diabetes. Check the patient's history, latest WCC and glucose. In either case, look vigorously for infection site (see p. 60).

3 Try to localize the source of infection. Don't forget to consider:

- Asking about abdominal pain, cough, chest pain, diarrhoea, dysuria/frequency, prosthesis/heart valves, rashes, rigors/chills.
- Recent surgery or invasive procedure?
- Recent sexual contacts, travel abroad (TB, malaria, amoebiasis)?
- Drugs

Common sites for infection:

- Chest, wound/line sites, bladder.
- Skin, leg ulcers.
- ENT (remember ears). Check for meningism.
- IV lines, catheters, drains—how long have these been in place?
- Do not forget to examine the genitalia, do a PR (ischiorectal/prostatic abscess), and consider PV (PID). Check joints for tenderness and swelling.

4 Consider other diagnostic possibilities (see Table 7.3). Check the legs, as DVTs are easily missed.

5 Investigations to consider:

- Urine dipstick and MSU.
- FBC ± white cell differential. C&E, CRP, ESR. Blood gases or pulse oximetry if you suspect a PE or pneumonia.
- Blood cultures.

Consider further investigations:

- Other cultures (sputum, stool, CSF, wound swabs, catheter tips).
- Radiology (CXR, AXR, sinus X-ray, US, CT scan, ECHO).
- Serology.

6 Management. Take cultures and decide whether or not to start antibiotics straight away:

- You should start antibiotics if the patient is immunocompromised or diabetic as these patients can deteriorate rapidly. See p. 60.
- If the patient is otherwise well, has a T of <38.5°C and is not immunocompromised or diabetic, you can usually prescribe an antipyretic and withhold antibiotics until you have test results (e.g. WCC). Have the nurses call you if the T rises and discuss with your senior if in doubt. Conservative management is usually appropriate for patients in the following circumstances, if their T is <38.5°C:
- Up to 24 hours post-op or following invasive procedures.
- Following blood transfusion (see p. 85).
- If antibiotics started in the past 24 hours.
- Paracetamol (1 g 4- to 6-hourly) is a good antipyretic. For fevers above

Table 7.3 Common postoperative causes of fever.

Day 1–2	Day 2–4	Day 5–10
Atelectasis +/– infection	DVT	As for days 1–4
Aspiration pneumonia	PE	Deep abscess formation
UTI	Wound infections	

40°C, prescribe tepid sponging and fanning.

• If SBE is a possibility you need to take three sets of blood cultures from different sites and at different times (3–6 hours apart). Do not start antibiotics before consulting with your senior, as starting antibiotics before a diagnosis is confirmed may prevent isolation of an organism which makes effective treatment much more difficult.

• Remember to make best use of your microbiology department. They are usually eager to help you.

The immunocompromised patient with fever

A patient is defined as immunocompromised if they: have WCC $<2 \times 10^9/l$, an absolute neutrophil count $<1 \times 10^9/l$ (neutropenia), are HIV-positive with a low CD4 count, are on high dose steroids or other immunosuppressants.

On the ward

1 Take a quick history and examination (see above) remembering:

• The patient can have weird organisms in weird places, including the CNS.

• Check *all* orifices.

• They can deteriorate rapidly (within hours). Seek senior advice early.

2 Investigations:

• Culture everything!

• If there is a central line, take peripheral and central blood cultures (include a culture from each lumen of triple lumen cannulae).

• Stool, urine, sputum, MSU and wound swabs, including from around the entry site of indwelling IV lines. Get advice from a microbiologist for special stains and cultures of sputum and stools for AFBs, PCP, *Cryptosporidium*, etc., if HIV-positive.

• Consider removing lines and culturing the tips (cut using sterile technique (sterile scissors, gloves) and send to microbiology in a sterile container). Discuss with senior.

• Re-check FBC for neutrophil count, platelets and Hb.

• C&E and glucose. Consider amylase, G&S, clotting, ESR, CRP.

• CXR (mobile).

• Specimen for serology if patient is new.

3 Commence broad-spectrum antibiotics once cultures are taken. Antibiotic policy changes rapidly, so check the latest protocol with a microbiologist or pharmacist. Oncology and haematology units usually have a written management protocol available. An aminoglycoside plus a beta-lactam, with or without extra anaerobic cover (metronidazole), is usual. Add flucloxacillin if a staphylococcal wound or line infection is likely.

Fits

Your aim is to prevent the patient from harming themselves and to end the fit as soon as possible. Most fits last less than 5 minutes and do not require active treatment, but prolonged fits require urgent treatment to prevent hypoxia and brain damage.

When answering your bleep

- Ask for a ward glucose to be done.
- Note the time you were called and rush to the ward.

Differential diagnoses

Epilepsy and omitted anti-epileptic doses

Drug or alcohol withdrawal

Hypoxia (fever in children)

CVA, sub-arachnoid haemorrhage

Infection or inflammation of the brain and meninges

Metabolic causes: hypoglycaemia or suprahyperglycaemia, deranged Ca, Mg, Na, thyroxine, urea, bilirubin (liver/renal failure)

Post-traumatic (sub-dural haematoma)

Drug overdose—tricyclics, phenothiazines, amphetamines

About half are idiopathic

On the ward

1 Place the patient in the recovery position. Protect the patient's head with a pillow.

2 Do not forcibly restrain the patient as it tends to prolong the fit.

- Give 100% O_2 by face-mask and insert an oral airway if possible, but never force one. The risk of choking on the vomit is less than that of choking on a tooth!
- Establish IV access using a butterfly needle. Get help if you are struggling.
- Give 5–10 mg diazepam (IV bolus) or rectal diazepam (10 mg) if IV access is impossible. If the fit does not terminate within 5 minutes of IV therapy, repeat diazepam 5 mg/minute up to

20 mg or until significant respiratory depression occurs.

- If not already done, check blood glucose with blood glucose stick. If the patient is hypoglycaemic (glucose <2.5) give 50 ml of 50% dextrose IV immediately. Flush the line with saline as concentrated dextrose is highly irritant. Alternatively give glucagon (1–2 mg IM or SC).

3 If the patient is still fitting, call your senior. Meanwhile, if the patient is not already dosed with it, give phenytoin 1000–1500 mg (15–18 mg/kg) IV slowly (not exceeding 50 mg/minute). Watch for hypotension. If the patient has been taking phenytoin, the next step is phenobarbitone (15–20 mg/kg IV slowly (up to 100 mg/minute) or IM)—but get senior advice first. The patient may need to be ventilated.

4 Once the fit has terminated:

- Examine the patient for localizing CNS signs, evidence of raised ICP (check fundi, BP and pulse).
- The patient will probably sleep deeply for some time.
- Consider consequences for the patient's driving licence (see p. 220).

5 Investigations to consider:

- FBC, C&E, blood glucose, liver biochemistry, Ca, Mg.
- ABGs.
- Blood cultures if febrile.
- CXR.
- CT scan if the cause is unclear and there are localizing neurological signs, papilloedema or head injury.
- LP if suspected bacterial meningitis (exclude a space occupying lesion first, preferably with CT. If unsure, ask your senior. LP in the presence of an obstructed CSF flow can cause coning).

• Toxicology screen if indicated by the history.
• Blood for anticonvulsant levels (some hospitals can do these within an hour).

Hints

• If you arrive after the patient has stopped fitting but it sounds like a typical grand mal seizure, discuss prophylaxis with your seniors. If known epileptic, consider why they fitted now:
Does it fit with their usual pattern of seizures?
Intercurrent infection.
Alcohol abuse.
Poor adherence to treatment.
• A useful alternative to phenytoin (especially for alcoholics) is a ready-mixed 0.8% clomethiazole solution for IV infusion; run in 40–100 ml over 5–10 minutes.
If you suspect malnourishment or chronic alcohol abuse, give thiamine 100 mg IV.

Intravenous fluids

If you have never done it before, prescribing IV fluids can look horribly complicated. It isn't, providing you keep an eye out for the cardinal sins of IV hydration:

1 Over-hydration, risking heart failure.
2 Electrolyte imbalance, especially Na and K.
3 Phlebitis.
4 Unnecessary and expensive if the patient can drink!

How to prescribe IV fluids

1 Decide on the daily volume of fluid required:
• Look at the fluid chart each day to make sure that you are keeping up with (and not grossly exceeding) daily losses. Remember that in addition to recorded losses (urine, faeces, vomit), people lose 500 ml/24 hours in insensible losses.
• The average person needs 2–3 litres/24 hours (each litre given 8-hourly).
2 Decide on which fluid(s) to use:
Most patients can be given a daily total of 2–3 litres of fluid in ratio of 2 litres of 5% dextrose water to 1 litre of normal (0.9%) saline. These should contain a total of 40 mmol of K and 60–120 mmol Na in 24 hours. This is typically written up as shown in Table 7.4.
3 Exceptions:
• Replace saline with dextrose water in patients with liver failure or ascites.
• Avoid dextrose water in patients

Table 7.4 Example of typical fluid chart.

Date	Time	Fluid	Volume (ml)	Signature
1/1/02	8 hours	Normal saline + 20 mmol KCl	1000	J. Bloggs
1/1/02	8 hours	5% dextrose	1000	J. Bloggs
1/1/02	8 hours	5% dextrose + 20 mmol KCl	1000	J. Bloggs

recovering from DKA or with hyponatraemia.

• Potassium imbalance is easy to achieve with IV fluids—and easy to correct. Measure electrolytes daily and adjust the K accordingly. If the K is suddenly very high, repeat the sample. Spurious hyperkalaemia can occur if you take blood from the drip arm, leave the tourniquet on too long or haemolyse the cells

• Hyponatraemia is a common and potentially lethal complication of IV hydration. If the patent's Na begins to creep below 135 mmol/l, the first step is to reduce the total IV fluid load and substitute dextrose with normal saline (see Hyponatraemia, p. 84).

Hints

• Patients with fever require about 10% more fluid for every degree Celsius above normal 37°C

• At least daily, examine elderly patients for signs of fluid overload and reduce fluids if necessary. Check the fluid charts and request daily weighing.

• See Table 7.5 for a rough guide to body fluid content.

Upper gastrointestinal bleeds

Always attend to GI bleed calls urgently as these patients can deteriorate rapidly, and apparently small bleeds can herald major bleeds. Most reported bleeds, however, are minor and do not require urgent action.

While answering your bleep

Ask for BP and pulse to be taken as you head for the ward.

On the ward

The basic approach for all upper GI bleeds is the same:

1 See the patient. Assess the severity of the bleed.

2 If the patient is hypovolaemic or at high risk for a major bleed (see box below) then they will require urgent treatment. To assess for severe hypovolaemia, check the BP, pulse and JVP (pulse >100/minute, sweaty and pale, cold peripheries, postural drop >20 mmHg and JVP imperceptible when lying at 30° or less).

Table 7.5 A rough guide to the electrolyte content and daily production of body fluids.

Fluid	Na$^+$ (mmol)	Cl$^-$ (mmol)	K (mmol)	HCO$_3$ (mmol)	Daily (ml)
Sweat	50	40	5	–	Variable
Gastric	60–100	100	10	–	1500–2000
Bile	140	100	5	15–30	200–800
Pancreas	140	75	5	70–120	200–800
Ileum	140	100	5	15–30	2000–3000
Diarrhoea	50	40	35	45	Variable

3 As usual, treat on the basis of clinical findings. Remember that a small initial fall in Hb could be associated with a massive life-threatening bleed.

High risk patients

Age <60 years

Melaena (altered blood passing PR, which can be due to a substantial *upper* GI bleed)

Severe bleed

Re-bleed in same admission

Patients on anticoagulant therapy

Co-existent cardiac, respiratory or renal failure

Known or suspected oesophageal varices or cirrhosis

High risk and hypovolaemic patients

If the patient is hypovolaemic or a high risk patient

1 Notify your senior immediately.

2 Remove false teeth. If hypotensive, give 100% O_2 and lower the patient's head.

3 Insert two cannulae (one in either arm), as big-bored as you can manage, even if the patient's bleeding seems to have stopped.

4 If the pulse is greater than 100 bpm or there are other signs of a major bleed, give 500 ml of colloid (Haemaccel) or 5% dextrose water as fast as possible and repeat if necessary while waiting for blood.

5 Urgently cross-match 4–6 units of blood. Use O-negative blood if the patient is still unstable after 3 units of colloid and a cross-match is not available.

6 Do FBC and clotting studies. Trans-fuse until haemodynamically stable (pulse down, BP rising and steady, warm peripheries, good urine output); 80% of bleeds stop spontaneously but 20% re-bleed.

7 Insert urinary catheter. Monitor urine output.

8 Consider inserting a CVP line, especially if the patient has a cardiac history or difficult venous access (consult your senior). Keep CVP in the mid to normal range (there is a risk of a re-bleed if the pressure is kept too high).

9 If the patient is anticoagulated at the time of the bleed, anticoagulation will need to be reversed. Discuss with your senior as to the best drug and dose to use.

Further investigations and ongoing medical management (discuss with your senior)

1 C&E. Bear in mind that urea is often raised due to blood in the gut, so look at the creatinine to assess renal status.

2 ECG and CXR in high risk patients. AXR is usually unhelpful in the acute setting.

3 Give IV ranitidine (50 mg tds) or equivalent. Switch to oral therapy as soon as possible, as it is much cheaper.

4 Monitor: pulse, BP, urine output (+/– CVP) hourly until stable. Slow the rate of transfusion once the pulse is less than 90 bpm and BP systolic is greater than 100 mmHg. Ask to be called if there are signs of:

- Re-bleed.
- Further haematemesis or melaena.
- Pulse rate rises (by more than 10 bpm).
- Systolic BP drops by more than 10 mmHg.

- Urine output is less than 20 ml/hour.
- The patient becomes confused.

5 Repeat clotting studies if patient has had more than 4 units transfused. You may need to give FFP (see p. 85).

6 Repeat FBC daily. Transfuse so that Hb >10 g/dl.

7 Daily FBC and U, C&E. Repeat G&S if necessary (if previous sample used up).

8 Ensure 2 units of packed cells are available for 48 hours after the bleeding has stopped.

9 Keep the patient NBM for 12 hours (longer if surgery is likely), and for at least 8 hours before endoscopy.

10 Ensure that the patient is on the next endoscopy list (usually the following morning) and that the endoscopist is informed. Obtain the patient's consent.

11 Discuss high risk patients with the surgical team, so that surgery can be arranged more smoothly if the patient deteriorates.

12 Consult with your team for further management.

Low risk patients

If after initial assessment the patient is well and at low risk of bleeding (e.g. only coffee-ground vomitus, no malaena, normal pulse, BP and JVP, warm peripheries):
- Take a history and examination to exclude the risk of a big bleed.
- Insert a cannula (just in case) and consider repeating a FBC and G&S.
- Inform your senior.
- Ask the nurses to monitor vital signs.

Most patients will require no further action.

Hints

- Confirm with the patient that they have had true haematemesis, not haemoptysis or an occult nose bleed.
- Vomitus can look like coffee grounds and contain small amounts of blood if the patient has not eaten for several days.
- In acute bleeds, the reported Hb lags approximately 12 hours behind the actual red cell loss. The minimum amount for transfusion is 1 U/g of Hb deficit; be guided by the clinical signs.

Lower gastrointestinal bleeds

Major lower GI bleeds, usually heralded by fresh or altered blood PR, are much less common in the hospital setting than upper GI bleeds, but can be just as serious. If called for a lower GI bleed, first exclude local causes such as piles and fissures and remember that major upper GI bleeds can present with altered blood PR. Follow the protocol for upper GI bleeds, with the possible addition of an urgent sigmoidoscopy. Discuss with your senior.

Glucose

You may be called for abnormal blood glucose readings. While *hyper*glycaemia is rarely an emergency, patients can die or suffer brain damage from *hypo*glycaemia so need urgent attention.

On the ward

Hypoglycaemia is usually caused by oral hypoglycaemic agents, poor insulin control and faulty ward glucose readings:

1 See the patient. If they are alert and well, repeat the blood glucose stick and take a sample for an urgent glucose test from the laboratory. Give them a concentrated sugar drink, such as sweet tea, and some biscuits.

2 If the patient cannot drink or is unconscious, administer 50 ml of 50% dextrose IV immediately. Flush the vein with 50 ml of saline, as concentrated dextrose is highly irritant. Also give 1 mg glucagon SC or IM.

3 Check the drug chart and recent insulin or oral hypoglycaemic doses. Adjust as necessary. Consider other, much rarer causes of hypoglycaemia in the hospital setting, including liver failure and acute alcohol consumption (which can and does occur in hospital).

4 Ask the nurse to repeat ward glucose readings. If the patient was semiconscious or unconscious, repeat hourly until stable. Ask to be called if ward glucose readings are lower than 5 or more than 11 mmol/l.

5 If the patient overdosed on long-acting insulin or an oral hypoglycaemic agent, set up a 10% dextrose drip and adjust the rate according to blood glucose readings (4–6-hourly once fully conscious and readings normal). Keep the drip running for at least 48 hours.

Hyperglycaemia is commonly caused in diabetics by acute illness, corticosteroid treatment and test error. Hyperglycaemia in non-diabetics may be caused by blood being taken 'upstream' from a glucose-containing drip; from latent carbohydrate intolerance which may be unmasked by sepsis; acute stress (e.g. MI)

and steroids; and from laboratory error. Be guided by the clinical state of the patient. Do not overreact to mildly elevated blood glucose (e.g. 11 mmol/l) on a single occasion. Hyperosmolar complications take days to develop, and although DKA can develop very rapidly, it has a dramatic clinical presentation, with decreased or absent consciousness:

1 See the patient. Repeat the blood glucose stick and also send blood for urgent biochemistry glucose analysis. Make sure the sample is not taken from a 'drip' arm.

2 Check urinary ketones. If positive do ABGs and manage as for early DKA. If negative and the lab glucose result is greater than 22 mmol/l, give an immediate dose of insulin (5–10 U Actrapid SC) and discuss a diabetic regime with your senior.

3 If the patient is diabetic with consistently elevated blood glucose, consider changing their drug management.

Hints

• Laboratory glucose results are 10% higher and more accurate than finger-prick assays.

• NIDDM may require insulin for control during acute illness (see p. 193).

Gynaecological calls

Gynaecological problems should be considered when investigating common symptoms such as abdominal pain and anaemia. If you are confronted with a complex gynaecological or obstetric problem, do not hesitate to refer to the specialists.

Vaginal bleeding

Menstrual bleeding is common in hospital, but if the patient is post-menopausal or the bleeding is abnormal, carcinoma of the cervix and uterus must be excluded.

Differential diagnoses

Menstrual bleeding (illness can cause abnormal periods)

Break-through bleed on the oral contraceptive pill, especially if the patient is taking antibiotics

PID, especially if IUCD is *in situ*

Fibroids or endometriosis

Tumours, especially cervical or uterine

Threatened miscarriage or ectopic pregnancy

On the ward

• Confirm that bleeding is vaginal and not rectal.

• Exclude pregnancy-related bleeding (ask about the LMP, contraceptive use and recent sexual history). Always think of pregnancy in pre-menopausal women. Send urine to the biochemistry lab for testing if the doubt.

• Consider PID, especially if low grade fever or tender abdomen. Do a PV examination for pelvic tenderness.

• Get a gynaecological referral if the patient is post-menopausal, or pre-menopausal with persistent bleeding and no obvious cause.

• Investigations to consider:
  • Pap smear.
  • FBC, clotting studies, ESR/CRP.

Hint

Anticoagulation does not cause abnormal PV bleeding but may unmask mucosal defects or tumours. Refer to a gynaecologist if the INR is within the therapeutic range.

Dysmenorrhoea

This is a common and painful problem for menstruating women.

On the ward

• Differentiate the pain from other causes of cramping, and lower abdominal pain. Most women will recognize period pain.

• Ask what medication works for the patient and prescribe this if there is no contraindication. Mefenamic acid 500 mg tds or ibuprofen 400–600 mg tds are useful. The side effects and contraindications are the same as those for all NSAIDs. Co-proxamol or codeine are perfectly acceptable alternatives. A hot water bottle also helps.

Haematuria

In the hospital setting, haematuria is commonly caused by UTI or catheterization. However, haematuria may be the first sign of serious renal tract disease, such as tumour or renal parenchymal disease (see Table 7.6).

On the ward

1 Exclude vaginal or ano-rectal bleeding (common sources of false-positives.)

2 Test for UTI: send an MSU and

Table 7.6 Differential diagnoses of haematuria (consider the anatomy of the renal tract).

Renal tract	Extra-renal
• UTI	*Systemic disorder*
• Trauma – catheters, surgery	• Bleeding diathesis
• Calculi	• Vasculitis (SLE, SBE, etc.)
• Prostatic disease	• Malignant hypertension
• Tumours	• Emboli
• Bladder inflammation (e.g. infection, recent surgery, chemotherapy)	• Sickle cell disease

Parenchymal disease
• Acute glomerulonephritis
• Cystic diseases
• Tumours
• Analgesic nephropathy
• TB

repeat the dipstick (look for blood and protein). If symptomatic (dysuria, frequency ± low grade fever) treat for UTI once the MSU is sent (see p. 105).

3 If a UTI is unlikely or the patient is unwell, discuss with your senior. Consider other causes (see above) and further investigations in light of clinical context:

• Urine cytology.
• FBC, ESR, CRP, C&E.
• AXR for calculi; urogram.
• Repeat urinary dipstick daily until diagnosis is clear.

Hints

• Urinary catheters can cause slight haematuria and usually do not require active treatment unless infection or non-trivial trauma is present.
• If the urinary dipstick reveals significant proteinuria (++ or more), renal parenchymal disease becomes more likely than a UTI. A very fresh sample of urine must be examined urgently for casts, etc. Commence a 24-hour urine collection to measure protein and creatinine clearance.

• If no red cells are seen on microscopy despite significant dipstick positive haematuria, consider haemolysis or myoglobinuria (rare).
• Anticoagulation within the therapeutic range rarely causes haematuria, but may unmask renal tract pathology. Repeat the clotting studies and discuss with your senior.

Headaches

Tension headaches are common in hospital. However, a severe headache with additional symptoms can be serious. The key to the diagnosis is the history.

Differential diagnoses and key symptoms

1 *Tension headache:* no associated symptoms. Pain can be severe, usually symmetrical and band-like.

continued

2 *Migraine:* usually history of previous episodes. Severe, throbbing pain which may be unilateral or asymmetric. May have prodromal symptoms (visual symptoms such as flashing lights, tunnel vision, cranial nerve deficit rarely lasting more than 1 hour, N&V, photophobia). Classic history makes the diagnosis, but exclude other causes if drowsy, neurological deficit or visual symptoms. A variant is *cluster headaches:* unilateral pain becomes severe around one eye which becomes red, swollen and watery. Episodes last up to 1 hour, and can occur several times a day.

3 *Sinusitis:* dull, unilateral or central frontal headache. Local tenderness.

4 *Drug-induced:* especially nitrates, digoxin, tricyclic antidepressants, benzodiazepines (the morning after).

5 *Meningitis, encephalitis:* photophobia, stiff neck, ± fever and rash. Requires urgent LP (if no signs of raised ICP or focal neurology) and antibiotics.

6 *Subarachnoid haemorrhage:* sudden onset of severe headache (like an explosion in the head) and meningism. Occasional atypical history (small leaks) mimicking meningitis. CT scan ± LP (showing red cells uniformly spread throughout the CSF).

7 *Raised ICP:* present on waking, often associated vomiting. May have blurred vision, raised BP, slow pulse.

8 *Brain abscess:* non-specific pain. Diagnosis requires index of suspicion and CT scan.

9 *Hypertensive encephalopathy:* always markedly elevated BP (diastolic >130 mmHg) and other signs of malignant hypertension (p. 70).

10 *Subdural haematoma:* elderly, alcoholic, head trauma.

11 *Acute glaucoma:* usually presents with a dull pain behind the eyes which the patient may describe as a headache. Early: mildly injected conjuctiva. Later: overtly red eyes. Urgent ophthalmology referral required.

12 *Temporal arteritis:* patient >50 years old. Subacute onset of frontal headache. Commonly associated with fever, malaise, myalgia, weight loss, unilateral blindness or other visual disturbance (indicating imminent occlusion of the ophthalmic artery). A typical history, tender temporal arteries and a markedly raised ESR establish the diagnosis. Temporal artery biopsy may be negative.

On the ward

1 See the patient. Briefly exclude emergencies (meningitis, encephalitis, subdural haematoma, subarachnoid haemorrhage, acute glaucoma, temporal arteritis) with symptoms and signs (see box above).

2 Do a history and examination. Ask the patient if he or she has had similar headaches before (consider tension headaches, migraine and sinusitis). If history is typical for a tension headache or migraine and if there is no evidence of fever, neck-stiffness, raised ICP, or temporal artery tenderness, then prescribe analgesia (see below). If, however, the headache is persistent, you should examine:
- Pupils and fundi (raised ICP).
- ENT (otitis media, sinusitis).

- CNS (especially cranial nerves).
- Gait (if history suggestive of space occupying lesion).
- Palpate temporal arteries for tenderness.

3 Investigations to consider:

If the history is typical for a tension headache or migraine, and there are no sinister signs, then no investigations are necessary. Otherwise consider (depending on clinical context):

- ESR, CRP.
- LP and CT scan, sinus X-ray.
- Temporal artery biopsy, but a negative result does not exclude skip lesions.

4 Treatment:

Once the rare but serious causes are excluded, 1 g of paracetamol 4–6-hourly prn is usually effective. If the patient is already on paracetamol, try ibuprofen (400–600 mg qds) unless NSAIDs are contraindicated. The next line of therapy is codeine phosphate or equivalent.

Hints

- Always consider meningitis in patients with fever and headache, although any febrile illness may have an associated throbbing headache.
- The scalp may be tender with tension headaches, migraine, temporal arteritis or shingles.
- Be alert to depression in patients with recurrent tension headaches or migraines.

Hypertension

Hypertension is common but rarely requires treatment in the middle of the night unless there is evidence of heart failure, malignant hypertension or severe renal disease.

On the ward

1 Re-check BP and pulse. Note previous readings. Make sure you use a big enough manometer cuff if the patient has large arms.

2 Exclude:

- Heart failure: raised JVP, basal crackles, swollen ankles, enlarged liver.
- Malignant hypertension: headache; confusion or depressed level of consciousness; deteriorating vision. Perform fundoscopy to check for fresh retinal haemorrhages, and dipstick urine for haematuria/proteinuria.
- Renal failure: check urine output and recent creatinine result.

If heart failure, malignant hypertension or renal failure, start to treat the cause and call the medical registrar for further management.

3 Otherwise, an elevated BP alone is seldom an indication for treatment. However, if the diastolic BP is greater than 130 mmHg, put the patient to bed and prescribe an oral beta-blocker (if no contraindication) or a calcium channel blocker and aim to reduce the blood pressure slowly over 2–3 days. SL nifedipine can cause a dramatic fall in BP, so do not use without consulting your firm's policy. Call your senior if there is no response within 1 hour.

4 If the patient is in pain or anxious (common causes of elevated systolic pressure), provide analgesia and reassurance as appropriate.

Peri-op hypertension (see also Surgery, p. 186)

Pre-op hypertension: Most anaesthetists will not anaesthetize a patient with a diastolic BP >100 mmHg. Discuss prescribing 10 mg of nifedipine PO or further sedation with the anaesthetist or your senior. Five milligrams SL nifedipine will reduce the blood pressure within 5 minutes and may be repeated. Ensure the anaesthetist is aware of the problem.

Post-op hypertension is often related to pain and will settle with adequate analgesia. If persistent, discuss with your senior.

Hints

• Do not treat hypertension for at least 48 hours following a CVA. Dropping the BP under these circumstances can cause brain damage.
• Raised ICP can cause hypertension and bradycardia (Cushing's reflex).

Hypotension

Hypotension is a common call, particularly post-op. Hypotension is seldom an emergency, but while on the phone ask how far the BP has fallen. A fall in systolic BP of >20 mmHg is significant and >40 mmHg (or a systolic BP < 80 mmHg) is an emergency (see The moribund patient, p. 74).

Differential diagnoses
Low blood volume (bleeding, dehydration)
Low peripheral resistance (post-general

anaesthetic, infection, vaso-vagal, anaphylaxis, drugs: ACE inhibitors, nitrates, antihypertensives)
Poor cardiac function (arrhythmia, CCF, PE, tamponade, acute MI, valve failure, myocarditis, cardiomyopathy)

On the ward

1 See the patient and repeat the BP. If well but feeling faint, vaso-vagal or drug causes (including general anaesthesia) are likely. Drop the patient's head and raise the legs. Check the drug chart and do an ECG. Observe.
2 If unwell, feel their peripheries. If the patient has cold, clammy peripheries, consider:
  • Hypovolaemia (bleeding or dehydrated: JVP down).
  • Cardiac causes (MI, arrhythmia: raised JVP. Check for irregular pulse, basal crepitations, history of IHD, chest pain).
  • PE (raised JVP, short of breath. Check legs for DVT, often no specific signs).
  • Anaphylaxis (wheezy, short of breath, new drug started).
If the patient has warm peripheries, consider:
  • Sepsis (JVP variable, fever). Check for source of infection (chest, abdomen, urine, skin, cannulae, surgical wounds). Exclude immunocompromise (see p. 60). Note that in some patients, severe sepsis may cause circulatory shutdown (cold peripheries) without going through a stage of vasodilatation.
3 Treat according to the cause. If hypovolaemic:

- Place the patient's head down.
- Insert large bore IV cannulae. Give rapid IV fluid.
- Face-mask O_2 100% (at least in the short term).
- Catheterize and monitor urine output.
- Consult your senior.

If cardiac causes are most likely:
- The patient may go into shock. Get senior help and do an ECG stat.
- Give face-mask O_2 100% (at least in the short term).
- Sit the patient up if it is more comfortable for them.
- Arrange for a mobile CXR.

If septic:
- Large bore IV access, rapid IV fluids.
- Face-mask O_2 100%.
- Blood cultures (two times) are mandatory, FBC, C&E.
- Consult your senior urgently before giving broad spectrum antibiotic cover.

Less common causes:
- PE. Do urgent ECG, CXR and ABGs. Discuss anticoagulation with your senior.
- Anaphylaxis. Give 100% O_2; adrenaline 0.5–1 ml of a 1:1000 solution IM/IV; salbutamol 5 mg nebulizer if wheezy; hydrocortisone 100 mg IV and chlorpheniramine 10 mg IV.
- Consider adrenal insufficiency, especially if the patient is on steroids or has a history of Addison's. Give hydrocortisone 100 mg IV (to cover the added stress of illness irrespective of the cause).

4 If you feel out of your depth, call for senior help immediately. Most often the cause is obvious but if not, do the following until help arrives:

- IV access.
- Face-mask O_2.
- ECG and mobile CXR.
- Bloods: FBC and clotting screen (INR and APTT); C&E; glucose; G&S (cross-match if suspect bleeding—see GI bleeds, p. 63); ABGs or at least pulse oximeter, and blood cultures.
- Monitor urine output and consider catheterization.

Hints

- Post-op falls in BP are common and often due to opiate analgesia. If the patient is otherwise well with no evidence of bleeding, ask the nurses to continue to monitor the T, BP and pulse and to call you if the patient becomes unwell or the BP substantially dips from its post-op plateau. The BP should rise as the anaesthesia wears off.
- Always re-check the BP yourself, remembering to use a big enough cuff for large arms.
- Bradycardia suggests a vaso-vagal or arrhythmia (e.g. complete heart block unless the patient is on beta-blockers or has raised ICP).
- If the patient is hypovolaemic, but there is no evidence of dehydration or bleeding, consider an occult bleed. Risk factors for occult bleeding include NSAIDs, stress ulceration, recent instrumentation/surgery, hidden fractures (especially in the elderly).
- Dehydration is common in frail patients.

Insomnia

Avoid prescribing sleeping tablets

without first considering why the patient cannot sleep. That said, it can be difficult to sleep on a noisy ward. Providing the patient does not take them home, short-acting sleeping tablets can be helpful.

Differential diagnosis and suggested management

1 Noise, light or too much daytime sleep. These are the commonest causes of insomnia in hospital and often the hardest to fix. Common sense suggestions include:

- Suggesting that the patient need not worry about not sleeping at night. If they really need to sleep, they will
- Avoiding stimulants before bedtime, such as cigarettes, tea or coffee
- Wearing ear plugs and an eye visor at night
- Ask the nursing staff whether it is possible to cancel the patient's early morning observations. Minimize noise from monitors
- Resolve conflicts between patients (consider moving beds around)
- Move the patient to a side room if possible, or to a quieter corner of the ward

2 Pain:

- Analgesia will facilitate sleep better than sleeping tablets

3 Confusion, excessive anxiety or irritation, depression:

- Do not sedate the patient without excluding medical causes such as hypoxia, alcohol withdrawal, wrong drug dosages or electrolyte derangements (check fluid and drug charts)
- Depression is common in hospital patients (see p. 110). Be wary of inducing benzodiazepine addiction in such patients (who may be especially vulnerable). Seek psychiatric and pharmacological advice if in doubt.

4 Disturbed sleep pattern due to frequency of micturition, orthopnoea or PND:

- The patient may need better control of LVF. Avoid prescribing diuretics close to bedtime

5 Disturbance in regular medication and bedtime habits:

- Often patients take an over-the-counter 'sleeping remedy' at home or have a supply of sleeping tablets which are not included in the GP's letter. The patient may not inform you about them unless specifically asked, and may suffer rebound insomnia in hospital
- You can prescribe patients a tot or two of liquor before bedtime if they are used to it—but ask your senior first!

Management with benzodiazepines

Benzodiazepines (e.g. temazepam 10–20 mg or oxazepam 15–30 mg) are the mainstay of therapy for insomnia but some patients cannot tolerate them. A useful alternative is chloral hydrate (500–1000 mg PO or PR) but do not use in patients with renal or hepatic failure. Amitriptyline 25–50 mg nocte is useful when chronic pain accompanies sleep disturbance. Use lower doses of all seda-tives in the elderly (consult the *BNF*).

If you prescribe a sedative, tell the patient to call the nursing staff if they need the toilet. Sedatives in an unfamil-iar environment can cause falls.

Itching

Except in the unusual event of anaphy-laxis, itching is rarely serious, but can be very distressing for the patient. Exclude simple dermatological problems before considering symptomatic treatment if the patient has skin lesions or a rash (see Rashes, p. 81).

Differential diagnoses (if no visible skin lesions or rash)
- Dry skin
- Drugs or allergies
- Jaundice
- Early shingles
- Infestations (scabies, lice)
- Rarities: polycythaemia rubra vera (myeloproliferative diseases)
              Hodgkin's lymphoma
              Late renal failure

On the ward

1 Check the patient's skin for rashes or lesions. If present, see Rashes, p. 81.
2 If there are no visible skin lesions, by far the most common cause of itching is dry skin, followed by drug reactions. Try to identify and replace the drug (seek pharmacological advice if unsure). Treat with emollient lotions after bathing (e.g. calamine lotion). Use cold compresses and moisturizers such as E-45 for local-ized itching. Advise minimal use of soap and shampoo. Discuss alternatives with nurses.
3 If you are called at night and the patient is well, it is reasonable to treat symptomatically. Choose a sedating antihistamine at night (e.g. chlorpheni-ramine 4 mg tds) or a non-sedating one if preferred by the patient (e.g. terfenadine 60 mg bd).

Hint

Scabies is common and can cause intense itching anywhere on the body except the head. The S-shaped burrows are easy to miss—look carefully around the itching site, particularly along the fingers and in the webs. Contrary to popular mytholo-gy, scabies does not imply that the patient is unhygienic. Consult the *BNF* for treatment of scabies and other infes-tations. Clothes and bedding need to be washed. Check with nurses that other nearby patients (or staff!) are not simi-larly infested.

The moribund patient

If you are called to see a 'flat' patient, don't panic. You usually have more time than you think. The priority is to buy time by supporting the vital functions while getting basic background informa-tion and examining as you go. Call your senior early and do not be afraid to call the crash team *before* the patient arrests. Think CASH (Table 7.7)! Stay calm and remain polite. Saying 'please' and 'thank you' when delegating jobs will inspire confidence and ensure that the team works efficiently.

Table 7.7 Differential diagnoses. (Acronym: CASH.)

Chest	Abdomen	Systemic	Head
Pulmonary oedema	Haemorrhage	Drug overdose, especially opiates	CVA
MI, arrhythmia	Perforated viscus	Hypothermia	Post-ictal
Pneumonia	Pancreatitis	Septicaemia	
Asthma		Hypoglycaemia	
Pulmonary embolus		Anaphylaxis	
Dissecting aneurysm		Serious electrolyte derangement or dehydration	
Tension pneumothorax			

On the ward

1 See the patient urgently. Check their ABC:

Airway clear?	Y/N
Breathing?	Y/N
	Trachea central?
	Bilateral breath sounds?
Circulation?	Pulse?—Y/N
	If Y—BP?

2 Bring (or get somebody to bring) the crash trolley to hand and to call the crash team if an arrest looks imminent.

3 Establish large bore IV access: 16 G if possible. Don't rush. Consider inserting two cannulae at separate sites.

4 Give O_2.

5 If BP <80 mmHg, consider starting a rapid colloid infusion (Haemaccel) unless a cardiac cause is probable. Use saline if sepsis is likely

6 While the infusion is being set up, quickly assess preceding symptoms, PMH and current medications. Examine the chest and heart.

7 If a cardiac cause is likely:
• Do an ECG and request a mobile CXR. Do not delay treatment.
• Pulmonary oedema, arrhythmias or

MI are the most likely causes. Consider pericardial tamponade.

8 Exclude hypoglycaemia or opiate overdose:
• If blood glucose is less than 2.5 mmol/l, give 50 ml of 50% glucose IV (flush vein with saline afterwards) or 1 mg glucagon IV/IM/SC.
• Note the size of pupils. Give naloxone 400–800 µg IV if the patient has pinpoint pupils and is on opiates. Repeat if necessary.

9 Listen to the chest. If markedly tachypnoeic in the absence of pulmonary oedema or pneumothorax, consider PE.

10 Feel the peripheries. If the patient has warm peripheries with hypotension, consider sepsis.

11 Consider anaphylaxis:
• New drug started recently IV, intravenous, NSAID, wheezy, swollen lips/eyelids, urticarial rash.
• Give 100% O_2; adrenaline 1 ml of a 1 : 1000 solution IM/IV; salbutamol 5 mg nebulizer; hydrocortisone 100 mg IV and chlorpheniramine 10 mg IV.

If the cause is not clear, do a brief neurological examination: level of consciousness (obeying commands), pupils and eye movements, limb tone, reflexes and plantars. Consider occult bleeding. Seek senior advice.

12 Urgent investigations:
- ECG.
- FBC and INR, C&E, glucose, amylase.
- ABGs.
- Mobile CXR, as erect as possible to check for free air under the diaphragm. View carefully for a pneumo–thorax, often missed in a panic.

Hints

- Metabolic acidosis, confirmed by an ABG, can cause tachypnoea. If the patient has metabolic acidosis and hypotension consider sepsis, ischaemic bowel or perforated viscus or pancreatitis and acute renal failure.
- Relieve a tension pneumothorax by inserting a needle or Venflon into the second intercostal space, mid-clavicular line.

Nausea and vomiting

Any acute illness can cause non-specific N&V. Be wary, however, of prescribing anti-emetics without also investigating the cause. If the patient is distressed it is reasonable to give an anti-emetic before examining them.

Differential diagnoses
1 Surgical conditions
Intestinal obstruction (adhesion, hernias, tumours) and peritonism (perforation, pancreatitis, etc.)

---

2 Medical causes
Local causes
Oesophagitis
Gastritis
Peptic ulcer
Central causes
Raised ICP (tumour, meningitis, subdural haemorrhage, etc.)
Migraine
Systemic causes
Infection (UTI, pneumonia, gastroenteritis)
Metabolic (organ failure, electrolyte imbalance—Na, K, Ca)
Drug reactions (opiates, digoxin, NSAIDs, dopamine agonists, chemotherapy)
3 Special causes
Pregnancy
Inferior acute MI

On the ward

1 Exclude severe dehydration (BP sitting and lying).
2 Rule out common surgical conditions—**intestinal obstruction** and **peritonism**.
3 Think about **medical causes** as above.
4 **Special considerations:**
(a) Is the patient pregnant? Do βHCG
(b) In the elderly, an inferior acute MI can present with N&V in the absence of pain. Do ECG and serial cardiac enzymes.
5 When there is **no obvious cause** after history and examination:
(a) If the patient had a single episode of vomiting without associated symptoms or signs, ask the nurses to observe the patient and monitor T,

BP, pulse and urine output. Dipstick the urine

(b) If the patient has persistent N&V or systemic upset, consider:

(c) MSU, FBC, C&E.

6 Further investigations to consider include:

- Ca, Mg, phosphate, amylase.
- ABGs if severe vomiting.

7 Management options to control symptoms:

The two most commonly used drugs are prochlorperazine: 25 mg PR or 12.5 mg IM and metoclopramide 10 mg IM or IV (caution in young women for dystonic reactions). Alternatives include:

- Cyclizine lactate: 50 mg IM or IV.
- Domperidone: 30–60 mg PR.
- Droperidol: 1–10 mg IV or IM.
- 5-HT$_3$ antagonists (e.g. ondansetron, granisetron) are very effective but are expensive and usually reserved for chemotherapy-induced N&V.
- Diphenhydramine counteracts extra-pyramidal side effects of phenothiazines.

Oxygen therapy

This section describes how to give O$_2$ safely, particularly to patients with COAD.

Methods of oxygen delivery

Face-masks (e.g. system 22 or Ventimasks) are good for the acute situation but can be replaced with nasal specs (see below) for longer term use. *Controlled percentage* face masks control the amount of O$_2$ the patient receives, and are graded 24%, 28%, 35%, 40% and 60%. You need to adjust the O$_2$ flow rate at the wall or cylinder, according to the rate printed on the mask—usually about 2 litres/minute for 24% masks and 15 litres/minute for 60% masks. It takes at least 15–20 minutes for blood gases to equilibrate after changing the percentage of inspired O$_2$.

Nasal specs are useful if the patient cannot tolerate a face-mask and for longer-term O$_2$ therapy. It is difficult to regulate O$_2$ delivery with nasal specs, so regular blood gas checks may be necessary. For standard size specs, a flow rate of 4–6 litres/minute is usual for achieving an inspired O$_2$ percentage of 30–40%.

For patients with chronic obstructive airways disease

Under normal conditions, the concentration of CO$_2$ in the blood is the primary stimulus of the respiratory drive. Some patients with severe COAD become insensitive to CO$_2$ levels and are dependent on low O$_2$ levels (mild hypoxia) to maintain their respiratory effort. If you give too much O$_2$ the hypoxic stimulus is lost and they will hypoventilate leading to CO$_2$ retention (hypercarbia). This can lead to CO$_2$ narcosis and death.

Therefore, when *non-emergency* O$_2$ therapy is required in patients with COAD:

1 Start with a 24% face-mask and measure the ABGs after 1 hour to ensure that the CO$_2$ levels are not rising. You need to find a level that achieves a fine balance between improving oxygenation and keeping the CO$_2$ at a safe level. Ask

for senior advice if the CO_2 level rises >1.5 kPa above the previous ABG level or rises above 8 kPa.

2 If the CO_2 level does not rise but hypoxia is still a problem, increase the oxygen to 28% then 35%, etc., repeating the ABGs an hour after each change.

3 If you cannot increase the percentage O_2, despite persisting hypoxia, because of hypercarbia, a doxapram infusion or mechanical ventilation may be necessary—discuss with your team.

In emergencies, use 100% O_2,* even when the patient is known to have moderately severe COAD (unless you know they are fitting from CO_2 narcosis!). Hypoxia kills quickly (within minutes) whereas CO_2 narcosis kills slowly (over hours). You will have time to check the ABGs if there is a history of COAD.

Hints

- Use a humidifier with O_2 if possible.
- Patients may be left on O_2 for longer than they need it. Always ask whether or not they really need it. The face-mask and straps are uncomfortable and can cause nasty abrasions and bruises to the face of patients on warfarin or steroids.
- Strictly, you are supposed to prescribe O_2 therapy on the drug chart.

Pulse oximetry

Pulse oximetry measures the percentage of blood O_2 saturation, and is not a direct assay of P_{aO_2} or P_{aCO_2}. It is not as trustworthy as arterial blood gases, particu-

larly in COAD patients, as they may retain CO_2 in spite of reasonable percentage O_2 saturation. Also, pulse oximetry will not reveal quite a low P_{aO_2}. Remember that the O_2 saturation curve for Hb is a steep sigmoid curve that starts to plateau around a P_{aO_2} of 9.1 kPa (70 mmHg). This means a patient may have a very low P_{aO_2} of 8.5 kPa and still have better than 90% O_2 saturation. If in doubt do ABGs.

Phlebitis

Phlebitis is indicated by pain and redness at IV sites, and is prevented by changing the IV site every 2–3 days (important if the patient has a structural cardiac abnormality or prosthetic valve).

Management

1 Remove the cannula and apply heat (e.g. damp, warm towel).

2 Elevate the limb.

3 Give mild analgesia if the site is very painful (e.g. a NSAID such as ibuprofen 400–600 mg tds).

4 Suppurative phlebitis is more worrying (pus at the IV entry site, induration, fever and enlarged draining lymph nodes). Try to express some pus and send a swab to microbiology for urgent MC&S. Prescribe IV antibiotics to cover *Staphylococcus aureus*. If the patient is well, flucloxacillin alone may suffice. Discuss local protocols with a microbiologist. Surgical drainage is sometimes required.

---

*In practice, unrestricted use of an ordinary (non-anaesthetic) face-mask will only deliver about 60% O_2.

Potassium

Hyperkalaemia

K greater than 6.5 mmol/l needs urgent treatment, but first exclude false-positives from old or haemolysed samples. Repeat the sample if in doubt. In the hospital setting, by far the commonest cause of hyperkalaemia is drugs.

> **Differential diagnoses**
> *Drugs*
> K sparing diuretics—spironolactone, amiloride, triamterene
> ACE inhibitors
> Excessive K supplements
>
> *Metabolic acidosis*
> Acute renal failure
> Diabetic ketoacidosis
>
> *Cell lysis*
> Massive tissue trauma
> Massive blood transfusion
>
> *Mineralocorticoid deficiency*
> Addison's disease

On the ward

1 See the patient. Repeat K and check their renal function (U, C&E). In the meantime, if the initial K was greater than 6.5 mmol/l:

2 Do an ECG urgently (look for widened QRS complexes and peaked T waves).

3 Give calcium gluconate 10 ml of a 10% solution IV over 10 minutes.

4 Do urgent ABGs. If acidotic, discuss with your senior. The use of bicarbonate (100 ml of a 4.2% solution) is highly controversial.

5 Give 10–15 units soluble insulin with 50 g of glucose 50% IV.

6 Set up a continuous 50% glucose infusion (50 ml/hour) with insulin according to 1–2-hourly glucose readings (insulin drives K back into cells).

7 Consider polystyrene sulphonate resin (Ca Resonium) 15 g 6–8-hourly PO or 30 g in methylcellulose solution PR. As this causes severe constipation, consider giving a laxative at the same time.

Hypokalaemia

In the hospital setting, hypokalaemia is usually caused by diuretics, inappropriate replacement fluids or taking blood from the drip arm.

> **Differential diagnoses**
> *Inadequate potassium replacement in IV fluids*
>
> *Renal losses*
> Diuretics
> Other drugs—amphotericin B, carbenicillin, ticarcillin
> Excess mineralocorticoid (tumours)
>
> *GIT losses*
> Diarrhoea
> Vomiting
> Intestinal fistulae, villous adenoma
>
> *Intracellular potassium shifts*
> Alkalosis
> Insulin and glucose administration

On the ward

1 See the patient. If the K is less than 2.5 mmol/l, or less than 3.0 *and* the patient is taking digoxin, you need to replace K urgently, as there is a risk of arrhythmias:

• Give 20 mmol/hour KCl at a concentration not exceeding 40 mmol/l (60 mmol/l in emergencies). Concentrated K damages peripheral veins. Never give bolus KCl, which can cause fatal arrhythmias. If a central line is available, 20 mmol/hour in 50–100 ml of 5% dextrose can be infused, but ensure that the infusion rate is monitored.

• Do an urgent ECG, looking for low, small T waves. Consider an ECG monitor. Patients with arrhythmias should be transferred to the CCU.

• Monitor K 4-hourly until stable.

2 If the K is between 2.5 and 3.0 mmol/l:

• Oral replacement therapy is usually sufficient (see below). However, if the patient is at risk for arrhythmias (e.g. recent MI or on therapy for arrhythmias), give cautious IV therapy (10–15 mmol/hour).

3 If the K is greater than 3.0 mmol/l:

• Give oral replacement therapy unless the patient is NBM or vomiting. Prescribe 80–120 mmol K in divided doses per day. There is a wide range of pills with varying amounts of K in each (see below). You can also advise the patient to eat K-containing foods such as bananas and chocolate.

4 Investigations to consider:

• Monitor K every 1–2 days.

• Do ABGs if you suspect alkalosis (alkalosis causes intracellular K shifts).

• Consider measuring Mg. Hypomagnesaemia is a common problem when hypokalaemia is due to chronic renal losses and may cause the hypokalaemia to be refractory to therapy.

A rough guide to calculating the total amount of potassium replacement required

In adults, a drop of plasma K from 4 to 3 mmol/l represents a total body deficit of 100–200 mmol K (depending on body weight). Each further 1 mmol/l drop below 3 mmol/l represents a deficit of an additional 200–400 mmol K.

Oral replacement therapy

K content of oral supplements:
• Slow-K   8 mmol K
             (effervescent)
• Sando-K   12 mmol K
             (tablet)
• Kay-Cee-L   1 mmol/ml
             (syrup, if the patient
             won't take tablets)

Hints

• Avoid Slow-K non-effervescent tablets, as they cause severe oesophageal and gastric irritation. Use the horrible tasting, but more effective, soluble effervescent tablets or syrups.

• In patients with normal renal function, it is difficult to overdose with oral K. However, DO NOT give K if the patient is oliguric. Consult your senior.

• Low plasma bicarbonate levels suggest that the patient has long-standing, intracellular K depletion. K replacement can take days.

• Contrary to popular belief, hypokalaemia secondary to vomiting is due to metabolic alkalosis (which causes intracellular K shift and renal excretion of K), not to loss of K in gastric juices, which contain very little K.

• Be careful in prescribing long-term oral K supplements for patients to take home. Make sure that the GP knows to monitor the patient's K, to avoid hyperkalaemia.

Rashes and skin lesions

The algorithm below is designed to help you make an initial diagnosis of your patient's rash or skin lesion. By far the commonest cause of new rashes in hospital is drug reactions, but psoriasis, shingles and other relapsing skin conditions can all flare up with the stress of illness. Dermatologists are usually helpful and keen for referrals. Seek their advice if in any doubt. Questions to ask are:

1 Are the lesions filled with fluid?
   No—go to the next question.

Clear fluid	(1) vesiculobullous diseases.
Pus	(2) pustular diseases.

2 Are the lesions coloured but not red?

Yellow	(3) yellow lesions.
White	(4) white lesions.
Brown	(5) brown lesions.
Skin coloured	(6) skin coloured papules and nodules.

3 If the lesions are red, are they scaling?
   No scaling:

Macular/flat	(7) vascular reactions.
Papular/ raised	(8) inflammatory papules/nodules.

Scaling:

No epithelial disruption	(9) papulosquamous diseases.
Epithelial disruption	(10) eczematous reactions.

Disease categories (1)–(10)

1 **Vesiculobullous diseases:**
   • Vesicles: Herpes simplex; shingles; chicken pox; tinea pedis, scabies; dermatitis herpetiformis; dyshidrosis.
   • Bullae: pemphigus; pemphigoid; bullous impetigo; erythema multiforme bullosum.

2 **Pustular diseases:**
   • Acne; folliculitis; candidiasis; rosacea.

3 **Yellow lesions:**
   • Xanthelasma; necrobiosis lipoidicum.

4 **White lesions:**
   • Tinea versicolor; pityriasis alba; vitiligo.

5 **Brown lesions:**
   • Macules—freckles and lentigines.
   • Papules and nodules—junctional or compound naevi; melanoma; seborrhoeic keratoses.
   • Patches and plaques—café-au-lait spots; giant pigmented hairy naevus.

6 **Skin coloured papules and nodules:**
   • Rough surface— warts; actinic keratosis; squamous cell carcinoma.
   • Smooth surface—condylomata acuminata; basal cell carcinoma; epidermoid cysts; lipomas; molluscum contagiosum.

7 **Vascular reactions:**
   • Blanching lesions—macular and diffuse erythema (toxic erythema, e.g. skin rash of viral illness); ur-

ticaria; erythema multiforme; erythema nodosum.
- Non-blanching (purpuric) lesions—the vasculitides.

8 Inflammatory papules and nodules:
- Papules—insect bites; pyogenic granulomas; cherry angiomas; granuloma annulare.
- Nodules—furunculosis ± cellulitis.

9 Papulosquamous diseases:
- Plaque formation—psoriasis; lupus erythematosus; mycosis fungoides; tinea corporis; tinea cruris and tinea pedis.
- Predominantly papular—lichen planus, secondary syphilis, pityriasis rosea.

10 Eczematous reactions:
- Atopic dermatitis; dyshidrotic eczema; contact dermatitis; others.

Diagnosing skin tumours

Melanoma
Itching; crusting; bleeding; change in size, shape or colour of mole; weight loss; satellite lesions

Basal cell carcinoma
Pearly nodule/ulcer with prominent blood vessels

Squamous cell carcinoma
Non-healing; crusting ulcer with rolled edge

Hints

- Generalized erythematous rash (± blistering) and fever should ring alarm bells as they may be associated with serious bacterial infections (e.g. streptococcal and staphylococcal).

- Take very seriously any new rash in people who are immunocompromised (e.g. HIV, high dose chemotherapy, leukaemia), as this could herald sepsis, which may be rapidly fatal.
- Similarly, take seriously a new rash in people taking medication that may cause agranulocytosis (for example, ticlopidine).

Shortness of breath

When answering your bleep

Ask the nurse to assess the respiratory rate, pulse, BP and, if possible, peak flows and pulse oximetry readings.

Differential diagnoses
Acute LVF
Asthma
Pulmonary embolus
Pneumonia
Pneumothorax
COAD exacerbated by acute illness

Rarely
Pericardial tamponade
Anaphylaxis

On the ward

1 See the patient. Check the T, BP and pulse and assess for respiratory distress (respiratory rate >30/minute ± cyanosis) and hypotension.

2 If the patient is hypotensive, consider: acute MI, large PE, tension pneumothorax, pericardial tamponade and anaphylaxis. Lower the patient's head and institute emergency treatment. Get senior assistance (see Hypotension p. 71).

3 If the patient is markedly tachypnoeic or cyanosed:
- Give O₂. Even if the patient has COAD, it is safe to give initial O_2 and reduce as soon as possible (hypoxia kills quickly, high CO_2 kills slowly) (see p. 77).
- Exclude pneumothorax with auscultation.
- Give salbutamol 5 mg stat using a nebulizer. Repeat as necessary.
- Examine quickly for acute pulmonary oedema (JVP, basal crackles or effusion). If present, sit the patient up, give furosemide (frusemide) 40–80 mg IV, diamorphine 5 mg IV slowly and an anti-emetic (e.g. metoclopramide 10 mg IV/IM). Consider MI or arrhythmia and do an urgent ECG.
- Request a mobile CXR.
- Do ABGs.
- Notify your senior. Get help early if the patient is deteriorating.

Important note: if you cannot distinguish between early pulmonary oedema, asthma or pneumonia (often difficult to differentiate), treat for all three (see [3] above). If there are no signs of heart failure or asthma, consider pulmonary embolus. Heparinize if in doubt (see p. 105) and confirm the diagnosis later.

4 If the patient is not acutely distressed: take a full history and examination. Do not forget to ask about chest pain or leg swelling, history of walking to the ward, and any recent changes in medication. Consider the differential diagnosis and treat accordingly.

5 Investigations to consider:
- FBC, C&E.
- ABGs.
- CXR (expiratory to show a pneumothorax better).
- ECG.
- Consider urgent ECHO if you suspect tamponade.

Hints

- Hypoxia can cause euphoria, so do not be reassured by an apparently undistressed patient. Be guided by the signs.
- A good way to assess respiratory rate is to breathe with the patient, as this also reveals abnormal breathing rhythms (not all dyspnoeic patients are tachypnoeic).
- Patients at risk for pneumothorax include those with a central line, pneumonia, COAD or asthma. Pneumothorax is easy to miss on CXR; ask for an expiratory film.
- Psychogenic SOB (hyperventilation) is suggested by peri-oral tingling, pins and needles, carpo-pedal spasm and especially alkalosis on ABGs. Treat by having the patient breathe into a paper bag.
- A fever suggests infection, but also consider PE or MI.
- Check for pulsus paradoxus (drop in BP of greater than 10 mmHg on inspiration), which suggests an acute exacerbation of COAD, asthma, or tamponade.
- If possible, take an ABG sample before starting the patient on O_2.

Diagnosing the important common conditions causing acute SOB
Acute LVF
Raised JVP
S3 gallop
Cold peripheries
Basal inspiratory crackles

continued on p. 84

Severe asthma
Pulse >120/minute, rate >30/minute
Pulsus paradoxus (BP drop >10 mmHg on inspiration)
PEFR <100
Rising Pa_{CO_2} (anything over 5 kPa is worrying in the face of tachypnoea)
Exhausted patient barely able to speak

Pulmonary embolus
DVT, pleuritic chest pain, pleural rub
RV strain: raised JVP, RV gallop
RV strain on ECG: prominent R waves in V1–V2 (common), inverted T waves in III and V1–4, deep S wave in I, Q wave in III (less common)

Pneumothorax
Chest hyper-resonant to percussion
Markedly decreased vocal resonance (a very useful sign!)
Decreased breath sounds
Often funny noises or clicks with heart beat during respiration

The sick patient

The following is a checklist of things that you should consider when seeing any patient who is very unwell (modify in light of the specific system involved):
1 What are the T, BP, pulse, respiratory rate?
2 Are ABC adequate?
3 Does the patient need:
  • Analgesia?
  • ABGs or pulse oximetry?
  • Baseline bloods?
  • CXR (mobile)?
  • ECG or ECG monitor?
  • IV access?
  • IV fluids?
  • O_2?
  • Senior opinion?
  • Urinary catheter?

Sodium

Hyponatraemia

Mild to moderate hyponatraemia is common in hospital due to excess IV (hypotonic) fluids. Hyponatraemia usually develops over days; replacement of Na should be cautious. More urgent treatment is required if there are neurological symptoms which range from lethargy to severe confusion or coma, but symptoms should not be ascribed to hyponatraemia if the serum Na is >125 mmol/l.

Differential diagnoses
Over-hydration with IV fluids

Renal
Thiazide diuretics
Nephrotic syndrome
Addison's Disease
Interstitial renal disease

SIADH
Malignancy
CNS
Drugs—chlorpropamide, cytotoxics, haloperidol, thioridazine
Pus in the chest
Porphyria

Others
Cirrhosis
CCF
Severe hypothyroidism
Following relief of small bowel obstruction

On the ward

1 See the patient and assess their fluid balance (JVP, fluid chart, chest).
• If dehydrated, measure urinary Na. If urinary Na >20 mmol/l with hyponatraemia, consider renal causes. If urinary Na <20 mmol/l consider other causes.
• If not dehydrated, is the patient puffy?
If yes, volume overload is likely but exclude nephrotic syndrome, CCF, cirrhosis and severe hypothyroidism.
If no, but the urine is concentrated (osmolality >500 mmol/kg or high specific gravity), SIADH is most likely. Look for the cause (see above).
2 Investigations to consider:
• Urinary Na, urine and plasma osmolality, U&E, liver chemistry.
• CXR.
• Discuss others with senior according to clinical setting.
3 Management: Treat the underlying cause. Urgent Na replacement is required if the patient is severely symptomatic and serum Na is less than 125 mmol/l. Seek expert guidance.
• If hyponatraemia is mild with no symptoms, and the patient is not dehydrated, treat by restricting fluid only. Start with 1 l/day, and reduce to 500 ml/day if there is no improvement within a few days.
• If the patient is dehydrated with impaired renal function, give normal saline (0.9%).

Note: beware of correcting hyponatraemia too rapidly. This can cause central pontine myelinolysis with irreversible brain damage. IV hypertonic saline (5% saline at 70 mmol Na/hour) is rarely required unless the patient is fitting or unconscious. Discuss with your senior.

Hints

• Hyponatraemia due to ectopic ADH secretion may be the first sign of a small cell carcinoma of the lung (oat cell carcinoma).
• SIADH can only be diagnosed if the patient is hyponatraemic *and* the urine is more concentrated than the plasma.
• Mild hyponatraemia is frequently seen in severely ill patients ('sick cell' syndrome) but rarely requires treatment.

Transfusions

While blood transfusions are common in hospital, always be alert to transfusion reactions. Remember to reassure your patient that all blood is tested for HIV and other viral infections.

Blood transfusions

For chronic stable anaemia, see Anaemia p. 40.

Remember that these patients have had a low Hb for a long time. Providing there has been no additional acute fall in Hb, transfusion is not urgent and is seldom needed in the middle of the night. Ensure any blood tests (FBC, iron studies, B_{12} and folate, blood film, Hb electrophoresis) have been sent before transfusion. Transfusion should be slow, to avoid causing heart failure.
1 Estimate the red cell deficit (1 unit of packed cells raises the Hb by 1 g/dl).
2 In general:

• Transfuse the patient to above 8 g/dl if they have a reversible cause of anaemia.

• Transfuse to above 10 g/dl if they have an irreversible cause of anaemia (e.g. myelodysplasia).

3 Check the patient's pulse, BP, JVP and chest for basal crackles as a baseline before transfusing.

4 The rate of transfusion will depend on the clinical setting and the presence or absence of heart disease.

• Transfuse slowly (each unit over 4–6 hours) in the elderly.

• Give furosemide (frusemide) 20–40 mg PO before the first unit and then with alternate bags if you are concerned about heart failure.

• If the patient becomes fluid overloaded, give furosemide (frusemide) 40 mg IV (do not mix in the bag). Repeat as necessary.

5 If the patient has had a previous transfusion reaction, give hydrocortisone (100 mg IV) and chlorpheniramine (chlorphenamine) (10 mg IV) *before* the transfusion. This is often necessary in patients who have had multiple transfusions.

Hints

• Do not transfuse a new patient with chronic anaemia without checking iron and TIBC, B_{12} and folate (see Anaemia p. 40).

• Do not transfuse blood through lines used for solutions containing dextrose, as this causes red cells to clump.

In the acute setting

1 Estimate how many units of blood the patient will need. In the acute setting,

the Hb level lags the actual red cell loss by 12–24 hours.

2 Packed cells have few clotting factors and platelets. Therefore, for transfusions of more than 4 units, check the INR and APTT, and add 1–2 units of FFP for every 4 units of packed cells.

3 Transfuse to above 8 g/dl. Re-check the FBC daily.

Hints

• In acute and subacute bleeds, the MCV is normal.

• Remember hidden fractures in the elderly. The thigh can conceal 2 litres of blood.

Platelet transfusions

Indications

• Platelet count $<20 \times 10^9/l$, or $<40 \times 10^9/L$ and the patient is at risk of bleeding (e.g. going for major surgery).

• Thrombocytopenia or dysfunctional platelets with active bleeding.

To order platelets, you only need to know the patient's blood group; a cross-match is not necessary. If the patient has had a previous platelet transfusion reaction (common), administer hydrocortisone (100 mg IV) and chlorpheniramine (chlorphenamine) (10 mg IV) before the transfusion. If the patient has had previous severe reactions, discuss HLA-matched platelets with the haematologist (they are very expensive).

Hint

Platelet clumping often leads to erroneously low platelet counts. Always ask the haematologist to confirm an unexpectedly low count by manual differentiation.

Transfusion reactions

Slow rising fever <40°C

A fever of up to 40°C is very common during transfusions. It is treated by slowing the transfusion and giving paracetamol (140 g 4–6-hourly) if the patient is otherwise well.

Severe reaction

If the patient has a rapid T spike >39°C at the beginning of a transfusion, a T >40°C at any time, an urticarial rash or wheezing and hypotension (anaphylaxis):

1 Stop the transfusion immediately. Send the bag and line to the lab for analysis.

2 Give the patient hydrocortisone 200 mg IV and chlorpheniramine (chlorphenamine) 10 mg IV stat.

3 If the patient deteriorates or becomes hypotensive, call for immediate help and give 0.5–1.0 ml of a 1 : 1000 solution of adrenaline IM.

4 Monitor closely (risk of shock and acute renal failure).

Urine, low output (oliguria/anuria)

Oliguria is defined as a urine output of less than 500 ml in 24 hours. The minimum urine output is 0.5 ml/kg/hour (35 ml/hour in a 70 kg patient). Urgent assessment is required for an output of less than 20 ml/hour, a daily output of less than 500 ml, or for painful urinary retention (see Table 7.8).

Table 7.8 Differential diagnoses of oliguria/anuria.

Pre-renal	Renal	Post-renal
Hypovolaemia/hypotension • Occult bleed • Dehydration • Cardiac failure	*Nephrotoxic drugs* • Aminoglycosides • IV contrast dyes • Penicillins • Sulphonamides • NSAIDs	*Blocked catheter* *Retention* Prostate, tumour, idiopathic
Reduction in arterial hypovolaemia • 'Leaky capillaries' • Septicaemia • Pancreatitis • Post-major surgery • CCF, liver failure	*Systemic diseases* SLE, malignant hypertension, etc. Interstitial nephritis	
Renal artery occlusion Emboli, aortic dissection		

On the ward

1 Check first for post-renal causes:
• Palpate the patient's abdomen for a distended bladder. Catheterize if the patient is in urinary retention. Remember to do a PR in men and PV in woman once the bladder is relieved, to exclude prostatic disease and pelvic masses respectively.
• If the patient is already catheterized, ask the nurse to do a small volume (100 ml) bladder washout to make sure that it isn't blocked.

2 Check for hypovolaemia and sepsis:
• Check BP, pulse, T and JVP.
• Assess fluid balance. Remember to include unrecorded losses (sweating, incontinence, etc.).
• Consider sepsis.
• If the patient is hypovolaemic, challenge with 500 ml IV normal saline over 30 minutes. If there is no urinary response, re-check their JVP and repeat the fluid challenge if it is low (and there is no risk of inducing CCF). In patients with poor cardiac function give 200 ml challenges. Consider a central line to monitor the CVP if the patient is acutely unwell.

3 Check for CCF:
• Oliguria indicates very poor cardiac output. Management should be discussed with your senior.

4 If you are unsure of the cause, get senior advice and do the following urgently:
• C&E and urea. A creatinine : urea ratio of less than 10 : 1 (i.e. urea disproportionately raised) suggests a pre-renal cause.
• Urinary Na. A urinary Na of less than 15 mmol/l suggests pre-renal causes; more than 20 mmol/l suggests renal causes.
• Urine microscopy.

Hints

• Remember to alter the doses of renally excreted drugs if the patient has prolonged oliguria. Patients with peripheral oedema may still be hypovolaemic.
• Never use K-containing solutions for fluid challenges, as the impaired kidney may not be able to clear K.
• In a patient with oliguria or anuria (with a near-empty bladder), catheters can be very uncomfortable. This is relieved by a bladder washout. A washout will also exclude a blocked catheter as a cause for poor urine output.
• If a catheterized patient has passed absolutely no urine for many hours, the most likely cause is a blocked catheter. Palpate for a distended bladder. If a washout does not clear the catheter, try replacing with a new catheter.

Basic emergency routine

• If the patient is flat or very ill, get help fast and don't hesitate to call the crash team if you feel the patient is deteriorating. Check ABC.
• Briefly check for the 6 'H's:
1 Hypoglycaemia,
2 Hypotension,
3 Hypovolaemia,
4 Hypothermia,
5 Hypoxia, and
6 Arrhythmias (Heart).

Check the BP (lying and sitting) and JVP, look for cyanosis and measure the respiratory rate. A good way to do the latter is to breathe with the patient. Do a blood glucose stick, ECG, pulse oximeter reading and consider doing a blood gas and rectal temperature. Check urine output.

• Ensure good IV access and consider a catheter and O_2. Monitor the patient's condition (quarter to half-hourly observations, ECG monitor, urine output) and do baseline investigations (see below).

• If the patient is well or stable you have time for a more thorough history and examination, although this does not mean a full CNS examination at 2 am (unless the problem is neurological!). For stable patients, urgent investigations are usually unnecessary and impede technicians' processing real emergencies. Before ordering new tests in the middle of the night, look at recent baseline tests and consider how new information will change management. If a test is not urgent but you don't want to forget it, write the card for the morning and write in the notes.

Chapter 8: **Death and dying**

Terminal care

About 65% of people die in hospital in the UK. Caring for dying people is stressful. Evidence suggests that medical students and junior doctors come to terms with mortality much younger than most people.

There are five elements to good terminal care: communication, pain control, symptom control, good prescribing knowledge and self care.

Communication

Breaking bad news

Breaking bad news is difficult but important. Contrary to popular opinion, people remember how bad news was related to them. While every situation demands a unique approach, the following may be helpful:

• If you are uncertain about how to start, talk to the patient's nurse. It is generally a good idea to ask nurses what they think the patient knows before seeing the patient. Take a nurse with you to the bedside.
• If possible, take the patient to a private room to tell them bad news.
• Have tissues handy.
• Try to hand your bleep to a nurse or colleague for at least 15–20 minutes.
• If you are unsure about how to proceed, it can be helpful to ask the patient 'What have you been told?'.
• Do not be afraid to give information. Studies show that people almost always want more information than doctors give them.*
• Watch and listen to the patient carefully for clues about how much information they want. If they indicate that they do not want to know everything at once, you may be more effective by feeding them information over several days.

> **Useful questions to assess how much someone wants to hear**
> 1 What have you been told?
> 2 Are you the sort of person who wants to know exactly what's going on?
> 3 Would you like me to tell you the full details of the diagnosis/results?
> 4 Do you want me to go on?

• Tell the truth and answer questions directly if asked (the patient may have been waiting all week to talk to you). Be ready to answer questions and to admit uncertainty. People are usually willing, even in the face of their own death, to cope with honest uncertainty. Have all investigations and findings to hand.

* In 1961, 90% of doctors thought that patients were better off not being told about terminal disease, compared with 3% in 1979. Martin J. (1993) Lying to patients: can it ever be justified? *Nursing Standard* 7, 29–31.

• Avoid using medical jargon.

• Write down relevant information and consider drawing diagrams to explain what you are saying more clearly (about 60% of spoken information is lost). Be prepared to repeat yourself many times.

• Ask the patient to write down questions they might have over the next few days. Give them your name or that of a colleague so that they can contact a doctor if they need to.

• Find out if the patient wants you to break the news to their relatives.

• Write in the notes what you have told the patient. This saves embarrassment for the team and sets a baseline for future explanations.

• Tell the nurses what you have told the patient. They can follow up with further information and support.

• Consider other people who can help with breaking bad news: other doctors, nurses, chaplain (about 25% of families accept chaplaincy support),* GP, nurse, police, social worker, support groups.

Ongoing communication with dying patients

• Pay a quick visit to the patient's bedside the next day (or at night if you're on call). Ask them how they're feeling and if they have any questions.

• Pain causes fear and anxiety, which may lead to the patient being withdrawn or depressed. If you are not getting very far with a patient, remember to ask if they are in pain, or if they are frightened that they might develop severe pain. Reassure them that pain can be con-

trolled; it is one of the most important contributions you can make to a dying patient.

• If someone's English is poor, ask the nurses or switchboard to help you to find an interpreter. Most hospitals have a list of employees who can interpret for you.

• Be alert to attention-seeking symptoms, such as headaches and insomnia, which are probably better treated with TLC than pills. A direct approach is usually the best one. A colleague once had a patient who had 22 symptoms in 24 hours and kept calling the nurses. The patient had been told that she had metastatic cancer that week. The doctor asked her outright 'How are you feeling about having secondaries?'. She burst into tears and told her she was terrified of dying—and stopped calling the nurses.

• Maintaining continuity of care, despite ward staff changes, is especially important for dying patients. Tell patients and relatives that you are going home for the weekend or on holiday, and the name of the doctor who will replace you.

• There are several stages of dying, including anger and denial. Pitch your information and communication to wherever the person is today. (This is easier said than done—remember to consider where you are at today too!)

• Do not be surprised by dying patients' aggressive or abnormal behaviour. This is when they need reassurance the most. Do your best not to take it personally—and check that there is no physical cause (for example, pain, hypoxia).

• Many dying people say that the most hurtful and distressing thing for them is avoidance and silence. Although it is often hard to do, allow patients to discuss dying with you (see below).

* Burgess K. (1992) Supporting bereaved relatives in A&E. *Nursing Standard* 6, 36–39.

• Look patients in the eye when you talk to them.
• Reassure people that pain and other distressing symptoms can be treated.
• Check that the patient does not have awful images of dying patients from films!

Five questions to ask dying patients

1 What have they most enjoyed in their life? Ask them to describe it to you.
2 What would they like someone to hear, that they have never said?
3 What would they most like to say to people they love that they have never said? Ask them if there is any way they can communicate this (for example, write a card, phone them from the ward, ask them to visit).
4 What are they most frightened of? You may be able to reassure them about pain and symptom control.
5 What do patients need to do (in practical terms) before they die? Talk to support staff (nurses, MacMillan nurses, social workers) and relatives about making this happen. It is very difficult for people to do things from a hospital bed.

Hint

Woolley and colleagues (1989) interviewed parents about their experiences of the way in which they were told of their children's life threatening illnesses. This article is well worth reading and pinning to your wall, as it gives an excellent, boxed outline of how to impart really difficult news. The reference is: Woolley H., Stein A., Forrest G.C., Baum J.D. (1989) Imparting the diagnosis of life threatening illness in children. *British Medical Journal* **298**, 1632–1636.

Difficult situations

• Try turning difficult questions for you back to the patient. For example, you can ask them: 'What makes you ask that question?'*
• If family members make it clear to you that they don't want the patient to know that they are going to die, ask your senior or nurses for help. The relatives are not your primary responsibility, although obviously you have to work with them. You can point out that it is your duty to inform patients of their condition.
• Write down relatives' concerns in the patient's notes.

Mistakes we've made: avoid them!

• Do not under-estimate how much caring for dying patients can affect you. If you feel irritable or low, don't give yourself a hard time.
• Avoid medical jargon.
• Do not overwhelm patients and families with big doses of information at once. Try to give information in bite-size chunks.
• Consider writing things down and drawing clear diagrams for patients to look at after you've gone.
• Do not leave patients waiting. If you

---

* Macguire P., Faulkner A. (1988) Communicate with cancer patients: Handling bad news and difficult questions. *British Medical Journal* **297**, 970–974.

promise to return, do so. People stay awake waiting for doctors to return.

• Never say 'Nothing can be done' or give the patient the impression that the medical staff have lost interest in them. Symptoms and distress can always be alleviated. Someone can always be present.

• Contrary to intuition, dying patients do not need to eat. It can be cruel to make them do so.

• Never give patients a 'date of death'. You will probably be wrong. Also, it is awful for all concerned if the patient lingers on after they 'should have died'.

Pain control
(see Pain control p. 133)

Pain is one of the things that dying patients are most afraid of. You can help them enormously, but you may need help:

• Use the pain clinic and ask for senior advice sooner rather than later if pain control is difficult.

• Remember the person may not admit to being in pain (check their pulse).

• Reassure patients that severe pain can be controlled, however severe.

Symptom control
(listed alphabetically in Chapter 7)

The *BNF* has a fabulous, two page section on symptom control in terminal care (look under 'Terminal care' in the index) which we have not tried to replicate for fear of being too quickly outdated.

Prescribing for the dying

• Many drugs are available as suppositories, which are useful if the patient cannot swallow or is vomiting.

• Keep drugs as simple as possible. Discontinue when close to death.

• Keep analgesia continuous. IV or SC opiate infusions are useful for this as are PRN doses to back up regular doses of analgesia. Nurses will usually set up infusions for you. In dying patients, the ultimate aim is pain control and quality, not quantity of life. Discuss pain management with the nurses so that they do not simply stop infusions to avoid respiratory depression.

• Consider PCA. Discuss with the ward pharmacist.

• Consider withdrawing IV fluids but discuss with seniors and relatives first.

• Infusion pump troubleshooting:
  1 Light not flashing—pump not plugged in; battery inserted wrongly.
  2 Infusion running too fast or too slowly—syringe incorrectly inserted, rate wrongly set, tubing kinked or blocked; needle site tissued.

Support for the dying and for you

Hospice (NHS or non-NHS); chaplain; hospital bereavement officer (if you have one).

CRUSE (widowed people caring for the newly bereaved), Cruse House, 126 Sheen Road, Richmond, Surrey TW9 1UR, Tel: 020 8940 4818.

MacMillan Nurses (nurses specially trained for palliative care), part of MacMillan Cancer Relief, Anchor

House, 15 19 Britten Street, London SW3 3TZ, Tel: 020 7351 7811.

Marie Curie Cancer Care, Marie Curie Memorial Foundation, Head Office, 28 Belgrave Square, London SW1X 8QG, Tel: 020 7235 3325.

Some questions to ask yourself if *you* feel excessively miserable caring for dying patients

• Make a list of five 'significant losses' you have experienced. Write down positive outcomes that arose from those situations, and identify ways in which you developed as a result.

• Do the same exercise for 'necessary losses'—those which you had no control over.*

Death

If the patient dies, don't panic. While really sad, death is often merciful when people have been suffering—for them, their relatives and ward staff. You can make a big difference to relatives if you handle the paperwork efficiently, allowing them to proceed with the funeral.

What to do when a patient dies

1 See the body.

2 Confirm death: fixed and dilated pupils, no respiratory effort for 3

---

* Hasler K. (1994) Bereavement counselling. Continuing Education article series (article 306). *Nursing Standard* 7, 31–35.

minutes, no pulse, no heart sounds for 1 minute.

If you are unsure, do an ECG or look at the fundi. The blood in the retinal veins separates into discrete blotches after death.

3 Write in the notes: 'Called to confirm death. No vital signs.'

4 Sign your name clearly with your bleep number. It is important that coroners and bereavement officers can contact you if necessary.

5 Note date and time of confirmation of death.

6 If possible write down the cause(s) of death.

7 NOTE WHETHER OR NOT THE PATIENT IS FITTED WITH A PACEMAKER OR RADIOACTIVE IMPLANT. If the patient is to be cremated, pacemakers and radioactive implants *must* be removed or they blow up in the incinerator at considerable cost to yourself. It is easiest to check for these while you still have the patient and the notes in front of you. If you do not check this now you will have to chase the body and the notes in the morgue in order to sign the cremation form.

8 Liaise with nurses about calling next of kin. Nurses usually tell the next of kin and meet them on the ward, but relatives may want to see you.

9 Note the GP's telephone number and name. You should call him or her at the earliest opportunity to let them know so they don't make a *faux pas* when they next see the relatives ('So how's so and so doing in hospital?').

10 Write 'GP informed' in notes.

11 Ask your senior early whether or not a PM is desirable, and what cause(s) of death should be written on the death certificate.

Telling relatives about the patient's death

1 Wherever possible, inform the relatives that their loved one is close to death. Ask relatives whether they want to be contacted in the middle of the night, establish the next of kin and how they can be contacted.

2 After death, ask the nurses whether they have told the relatives about the patient's death. They will often do so — sometimes before you make it to the ward.

3 If it is up to you to inform relatives, make sure you contact the patient's designated 'next of kin'. Ask the nurses who this is, or look in the nursing or medical notes.

4 It is usually best to tell the next of kin what has happened over the phone (rather than just asking them to come in urgently). Sometimes people don't want to see the body or would rather wait until morning.

5 If you receive the relatives, take them to a private room. If they have come a long way they might be grateful for a cup of tea.

6 Try to establish:
- If the body is to be cremated or buried. If the former, you will need to fill out a cremation form (see below).
- If the relatives will consent to a post mortem (see below).

Post mortems

- Preferably before the patient dies, ask your colleagues if they want a PM so that you can ask the relatives when the patient dies.

- PMs requested by the coroner are mandatory by law. Otherwise, you cannot force a next of kin to agree to a PM. Many people will oblige if you explain why you want one, particularly if it is a limited PM.

- Send case notes (complete with recent investigation results), the next of kin's consent form and a brief synopsis of the patient's history and hospital progress to the PM room, together with your name and bleep number.

- Request that the pathologist bleeps you or your senior with the results.

Death certificates

Only doctors who have seen the patient within 14 days before death are legally allowed to sign a death certificate. The next of kin must take this to the Registrar of Births and Deaths within 5 days (8 days in Scotland) in a sealed envelope. Give the signed death certificate to either the nurses, the ward clerk or the family.

If there is no next of kin, you must ensure that the death certificate is sent to the registrar.

Writing the death certificate

Make sure you fill in the death certificate correctly or you may be recalled by the registrar and delay the funeral. (Don't be too hard on yourself if you do make mistakes, as it is not the simplest document to fill out.)

1 Part one: Fill in the sequence of conditions that caused the patient's death. *1a)* is the condition that caused death. Causes of death are recognized pathological states, such as MI. The cause of

death must not be too general. For example, organ failure is not an acceptable cause. Other unacceptable causes are tabulated below. Ask your senior or ring the registrar if you are unsure about how to describe the cause of death.

Unacceptable 'causes' of death	
Asphyxia	Hepatic failure
Asthenia	Hepatorenal failure
Brain failure	Kidney failure
Cachexia	Renal failure
Cardiac arrest	Respiratory arrest
Cardiac failure	Shock
Coma	Syncope
Debility	Uraemia
Exhaustion	Vagal inhibition
Heart failure	Vaso-vagal attack

1b) and c) are diseases underlying this condition. For example, if the cause of death was MI, the underlying disease might be ischaemic heart disease, or chronic hypertension.

2 Part two: Fill in other diseases which were not directly linked with the cause of death in 1a), but which may have contributed to the patient's overall demise.

3 Sign the death certificate on the relevant part of the form.

4 Print your name, hospital and most recent medical qualification on the relevant part of the form.

5 Print the name of the patient's consultant on the relevant part of the form.

6 Fill in the counterfoil ('cheque-butt') part of death certificate. This retains the basic details of the death when the relatives have taken the main certificate.

7 Fill in the 'note to informant'. This is given to the next of kin.

• If you are unsure about any part of the death certificate, call the registrar's officer or talk to a colleague or bereavement officer. The registrar's office is in the phone book under 'Registrar of Births and Deaths'.

• Do not use abbreviations on the death certificate.

• If your hospital has a bereavement officer, he or she will usually discuss the request for a PM with the relatives and will help you with the death certificate.

• It is courteous to relatives to write the cause of death in lay-language (for example, 'stroke' as well as cerebral infarction).

• If your patient was a war pensioner or serviceman/woman, you can influence whether or not their spouse continues to receive war widow(er)'s pension by what you write on the death certificate. This is especially important if the person died from war-related causes.

• Doctors must record diseases which may have been due to previous employment.

Referring to the coroner (Scotland: procurator fiscal)

1 To contact your local coroner or procurator, ask your senior, switchboard, the police station or directory enquiries for the phone number.

2 It is the statutory obligation of the Registrar of Births and Deaths, not you, to report suspect deaths to the coroner or procurator fiscal. However, it saves time if you know what these are and can send the death certificate directly to the coroner. They are:

- Unknown cause of death.
- The patient was not seen by certifying doctor within 14 days of death.
- Death was caused by medical treatment (for example, dying in theatre, or within 24 hours of an anaesthetic).
- Death was suspicious in any way.
- Death occurred within 24 hours of admission to hospital without a firm diagnosis being made.
- Death was caused by a road traffic accident, an industrial disease or accident, a domestic accident, violence, neglect, abortion, suicide or poisoning (including acute alcohol ingestion).
- Death occurred during legal custody.
- Where there is any claim for negligence against medical or nursing staff.
- Death may have occurred from industrial injury or employment.
- Death of a foster child, patient under Mental Health Act (1983), mentally disabled people, Service Pensioners.

3 The coroner can request:
- The issue of a normal death certificate.
- A PM.
- An inquest.

House Officers rarely have to deal with this. If in doubt, phone the coroner and discuss the case.

Cremation forms and fees

You receive approximately £40 for every cremation form you fill out. 'Crem forms' are legal documents to establish beyond any doubt the deceased's identity, as incinerated bodies cannot be exhumed. If you have not seen the patient since death, you must pay a quick visit to the cold room so that you know you are signing the form for the right person.

Crem forms are straightforward to fill out, provided you are certain there are no radioactive or pacemaker implants in the body.

- Ensure you fill in the same cause(s) of death on the crem form that you did on the death certificate or you will be chased by the coroner.
- If in doubt, call the coroner's office or ask a medical colleague.
- If the family is poor you can forgo the crem fee. In some hospitals this is standard policy. If you choose not to accept crem fees, you need a tax exemption form from the morgue director or bereavement officer so that you don't get taxed for fees you haven't taken.
- Keep details of cremation fees you have taken as you need to declare them in your tax forms. Increasingly the Inland Revenue is checking up on doctors for non-declaration (see p. 209).

To check for pacemakers

- Feel the chest.
- Look through the notes for history of implantation of pacemaker or radioactive implant.
- Look for ECGs that will demonstrate an active pacemaker by small, regular vertical lines throughout the trace.
- The only sure-fire way to exclude a pacemaker is to see a recent chest X-ray. Make sure you see it before the radiology department removes it from the inpatient file.

Did you know:
- About 650 000 people die in the UK each year.
- At least 1 500 000 people suffer major bereavement each year.
- There are 3 200 000 widows and 750 000 widowers: one woman in seven is a widow, one man in 28 is a widower.
- 180 000 children under 16 have lost a parent (Office of Population Censuses & Surveys and from DSS Statistics Office, Newcastle-Upon Tyne).

Further reading

There are many excellent books and articles on death and dying. Ask your librarian. Here are some useful articles for starters:

Buckman R. (1992) *How to Break Bad News. A Guide for Health Care Professionals*. Papermac, London.

Continuing Education article series on bereavement counselling. (1994) *Nursing Standard*.

Cooke M., Cooke H., Glucksman E. (1992) Management of sudden bereavement in the accident and emergency department. *British Medical Journal* **304**, 1207–1209.

Egan G. (1990) *The Skilled Helper. A Systematic Approach to Effective Helping*. 4th edn. Brookes-Cole, Pacific Grove CA.

Macguire P., Faulkner L. (1988) Communicate with cancer patients: handling bad news and difficult patients. *British Medical Journal* **297**, 907–909.

McLauchlan C. (1990) Handling distressed relatives and breaking bad news. *British Medical Journal* **301**, 1145–1149.

Raphael B. (1984) *The Anatomy of Bereavement*. Hutchinson, London.

Thayre K., Hadfield-Law L. (1993) Never going to be easy: Giving bad news. RCN Nursing Update; Continuing Education article series. *Nursing Standard* **8**, 3–13.

Worden W. (1991) *Grief Counselling and Grief Therapy. A Handbook for the Mental Health Practitioner*. 2nd edn. Springer, London.

Chapter 9: **Drugs**

Don't worry if pharmacology seems a long time ago. Prescribing and giving drugs is not difficult.

General

• The most useful pharmacology tip is: *always refer to the BNF if in any doubt about any drug.* As a House Officer, you will rarely be expected to prescribe drugs that are not in the *BNF*. Also, read the *BNF* for entertainment during long ward rounds; it contains lots of useful information. For example, it contains prescribing guidelines for the elderly, the terminally ill and children.

• Make the most of your ward pharmacist. Not only are pharmacists happy to discuss patient management and find alternatives for problematic drugs (or patients) but they are often willing to find recent articles and other information about specific drugs for you. This can be useful for clarifying unusual side effects and for academic talks.

• For easy reference, make yourself a chart of common drugs and doses used on the wards and stick it on the front of your folder or notes. It is particularly useful to do this for infusion dosages, which can be painstaking to look up every time you make up an infusion. We have refrained from providing such lists in this book because every hospital's protocol is different and drug doses vary over time. As always, check the *BNF*.

Prescribing drugs

Drug charts

Drug charts are straightforward to fill out. Basically, there are three parts to a drug chart:
1 A place for regular drugs.
2 A place for 'PRN' or 'when required' drugs.
3 A place for one-off drugs.
For each section of the chart, you need to fill in the date, the generic name of each drug, its dose, how frequently it should be prescribed, and your signature. Abbreviations for prescribing are shown in Table 9.1.

Tips for filling in drug charts

• Write legibly. Other people have to administer drugs that you prescribe.

• In particular, take care in writing dose amounts and units. Micrograms (abbreviated mcg) can easily be mistaken for milligrams (mg); the *BNF* advises that 'micrograms' and 'units' be written in full. (A doctor was sued when a patient was given 125 mg of digoxin by a nurse who misread the scrawled 'mcg'. She had to open many packets of the drug to give such a dose, so also ended up in the dock for failure of common sense.)

• Develop a good relationship with the ward pharmacist. He or she reviews all drug charts and will bleep you if you prescribe anything idiotic. Similarly,

Table 9.1 Abbreviations for prescribing drugs.

Abbreviation	Meaning
ac (ante cibum)	before food
pc (post cibum)	after food
bd (bis die)	take twice daily
mane	take in the morning
nocte	take in the evening
od	take once daily
prn (pro re nata)	take when required
qds	take four times a day
stat	take straight away
tds	take three times a day
T. T.T. T.T.T.	one tablet two tablets three tablets
x/7, y/52, z/12	x days, y weeks, z months

nurses, who administer many drugs, will usually let you know if you have made a prescription error.

• Hospital pharmacists usually use green ink. To avoid confusion, use a different colour when writing on drug charts.

• If drug administration is complicated, write additional instructions on the drug chart. There is no harm in writing extra notes to nurses and doctors on the drug chart. In fact it is legally advisable to do so.

Writing prescriptions

Pre-registration House Officers are only permitted to write prescriptions for the hospital pharmacy. However, if you do need to write a prescription on plain paper the essential ingredients are:

• Date.
• Name of patient.
• Address of patient.
• Generic drug name and amount.
• Dose/day.
• Your signature.

For example:

> 27/8/02
> Mr JS
> 17 SWP Road
> Oxford OX1
> Carbimazole 10 mg bd
> (signature and printed name)

Controlled drugs

Prescriptions for take-home controlled drugs have to be written in a particular way, otherwise the pharmacy will send the prescription back. This wastes a spectacular amount of time. To write a controlled drug prescription:

• The prescription must be in your handwriting—don't use sticky labels.
• Include:
  • Date.
  • Name of patient.
  • Address of patient.
  • Generic drug name and amount (for example, '10 mg').
  • Dose/day
  • Number of tablets in **both** numbers and letters (for example, '10/ten tablets').
  • Your signature and printed name.

For example:

5/4/02
Mr TSD
2 Tatelman Street
Wolfchester WC5

MST continuous tablets 10 mg
10/ten tablets
10 mg twice daily for 5 days

(Your signature and printed name)

Verbals

In many hospitals you can prescribe drugs for patients 'verbally' over the phone to nurses. Typical verbal requests might be 'Mr Smith has a headache. Could he have two paracetamol please?' The nurse writes your prescription in the drug chart, with a small note saying 'Dr X will sign this'. Verbals are great for relatively harmless drugs, such as one-off doses of paracetamol or aspirin, or for doses of necessary drugs when you have been held up and coming to the ward is monumentally inconvenient.

• Check hospital policy. Increasingly verbals are not allowed by Trusts.

• It is important to sign verbal requests on the drug chart as soon as possible. Should any problems arise in the interim, the nurse who took the verbal is liable for damages. Because of this, some nurses refuse to take verbals and insist you come to the ward to sign the drug before it is given.

• Nurses will usually refuse to accept verbals if they think the patient should be seen by a doctor before taking the drug. While this can be frustrating, remember that nurses' scruples provide a big safety net for you. Everyone remem-

bers times when they were glad that nurses forced them to question what they were doing.

• Many hospitals allow a limited number of drugs (e.g. paracetamol, sublingual nitrate, lactulose, antacids) to be prescribed by nurses after calling the duty doctor. While you need not see the patient, it is prudent to check the reasons for the request. You may be required (depending on local policy) to sign for the drugs later.

Giving drugs

Nurses give oral drugs, suppositories, SC and IM drugs. In some hospitals nurses also give IV drugs. Usually the House Officer makes up infusions and may give IV drugs.

• Use a metal file to open difficult glass drug vials by scratching the neck with the file, and snapping it off. Nurses usually have a file stashed somewhere on the ward.

• Wear gloves or use your non-dominant hand when opening multiple vials. Your dominant hand's index finger can get chaffed with minute glass splinters if you snap open many glass vials consecutively.

• Avoid using normal saline as a dilutant for drugs in patients with liver failure; 5% dextrose is usually adequate.

Avoid dextrose in patients with diabetic coma. Give normal saline instead. Refer to the *BNF* for alternative dilutants for different drugs.

• When making up cytotoxic drugs, always wear gloves, apron and goggles (and keep your mouth closed!) Wash your hands afterwards.

Drug infusions

Continuous infusions are easy to make up, but they are a complete pain at 4 am. Always make up midnight infusions before going to bed. This is particularly true of morphine, dopamine and GTN infusions, which you will be called out of bed for otherwise.

To make up an infusion

1 Find the vial of drug in the drug cupboard. Check the dosage and the expiry date.

2 Open the vial (use a file if difficult — see above).

3 Draw up the drug into a suitably large syringe, usually 50 ml.

4 Draw into the syringe the required amount of dilutant fluid. Usually normal saline, water for injections or 5% dextrose, drawn from unopened (sterile) containers.

5 Label the syringe with a large sticky. Specify on the sticky:
- Date and time you made infusion up.
- Name of patient.
- Amount of drug in amount of dilutant (for example, 50 mg GTN in 50 ml normal saline).
- Rate at which solution should run (for example, 2 ml/hour).
- Your signature.

6 If the infusion is not needed for a few hours, put it in the fridge and let the nurses know where it is.

Prescribing drug infusions

1 Prescribe infusions on the fluid section of the drug chart. In some hospitals this is a separate sheet at the end of the patient's bed.

2 Write: a units of b drug in x ml of y dilutant to run at z ml/hour.

For example, 25 000 units of heparin in 50 ml N/saline. Run at 2 ml/hour.

3 To avoid confusion, convert the amount of drug/hour to the amount of infusion to be given every hour (i.e. ml/hour, not mg/hour). To do this, ask yourself the following questions:
- How many units of drug should the patient get per hour?

   For example, 1000 units heparin/hour.
- How many units of drug are there per ml of infusion?

   For example, 25 000 units/50 ml infusion = 500 units/ml.
- Therefore, how many ml do I need to give so that the patient gets the right amount of units per hour?

   For example, 1000 units/hour ÷ 500 units/ ml = 2 ml/hour.

4 You can always write additional instructions on the drug chart regarding infusion administration.

For example, 50 mg GTN in 50 ml N/saline; run at 1–10 ml/hour titrated against chest pain.

Administering infusions

If the nurses are willing to administer infusions, all you have to do is let them know that you have made up the infusion, and where they can find it.

- Otherwise, get a nurse to show you how to set up a pump (for example, Vickers). It is not difficult. Basically you insert the syringe into the pump with the drug label facing outwards, set the rate on the machine, plug it in and turn it on. You also have to remember to connect the patient to the syringe.

• Infusions can run through central or peripheral lines. Many infusions can run concurrently with other drugs through three-way taps or multiple-tap ('traffic light') giving sets. These are simple to set up with initial nurse supervision.
• Some infusions cannot be mixed with others. The most problematic are those containing chelating ions, such as Ca. Unfortunately these require a second Venflon or need flushing with heparinized saline (Hepsal) or saline before another drug is administered through the same line.
• Place the syringe driver below the level of the patient's head to avoid the risk of siphoning.

Intravenous drugs

If you are in a hospital where nurses do not administer IV drugs then you need to mix them with dilutant and give them yourself. This means doing an IV drug round 3 to 4 times daily.
1 Ensure the patient really needs the drug IV. Most drugs may be given PO, PR, SC or IM. It is time consuming for you and expensive for the NHS to give drugs IV.
2 Read the instructions in the drug packet. Some drugs can be injected directly into the patient's vein. However, they usually need to be diluted first.

Liquid drugs not requiring dilution

If the drug can be given without dilution, draw it up with a small syringe and inject it over the recommended time. Some drugs must be given slowly to avoid anaphylaxis or pain in the patient's arm which they won't thank

you for. Most drugs can be given quite quickly (over less than 30 seconds to 1 minute). Read the *BNF* and the drug's instructions.

Liquid drugs requiring dilution

If the drug comes in liquid form which needs diluting, this is easily done by drawing the drug into a suitably large syringe (for example, 10 or 20 ml), and then drawing in sterile saline or water for injection (available in small, sterile vials in the drug cupboard).

Always use sterile fluid when diluting drugs; patients can get septic from once-sterile fluid that has been lying around unsealed.

Powdered drugs

If the drug comes in a vacuum container as a powder, you need to dissolve it with a solute, such as water for injection. Most antibiotics come this way. To avoid giving yourself and the ward a drug shower (Fig. 9.1):
1 Draw the required amount of water for injection into a suitably large syringe through a needle. Tap or push the end of the syringe to expel any air, so that the water is flush with the top of the syringe.
2 Remove the flip-off plastic top of the drug vial.
3 Push the needle through the rubber top of the drug vial and withdraw some air to create a vacuum inside the vial.
4 Tap or tilt the syringe so that the withdrawn air moves through the water to the back of the syringe.
5 Inject the water into the vial, with the assistance of the vacuum you have just

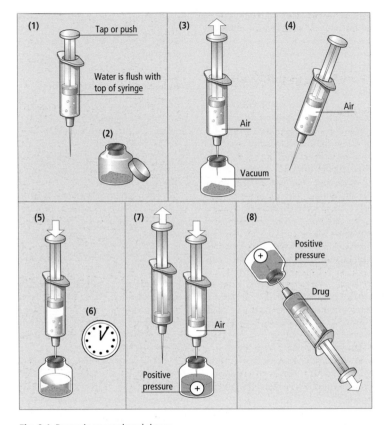

Fig. 9.1 Preparing powdered drugs.

created. You may need to repeat this several times.

6 When you have injected enough water, shake the vial (or leave it to dissolve while you do something else).

7 Withdraw the needle. Draw some air into the syringe. Re-introduce the needle into the vial through the rubber top and inject some air to create positive pressure inside the vial.

8 Turn the vial upside down and withdraw the dissolved drug from the vial with the assistance of the positive pressure.

9 Don't worry if on first attempts you spray yourself, the desk and unwary

passers-by with the drug. You will soon be able to do the whole thing perfectly in your sleep.

Specific drug topics

Antibiotics

• Check your hospital drug guidelines with seniors and pharmacologists. Each hospital has particular protocols which are usually published.
• Always ask patients if they have known antibiotic (penicillin) allergy before prescribing penicillin or cephalosporin antibiotics. Erythromycin is a reasonable alternative to ampicillin and related drugs. Also be alert to pseudomembranous colitis (send stool specimen for *Clostridium difficile*) if the patient develops diarrhoea and fever.
• Common antibiotic side effects include diarrhoea and vaginal (and other) candidiasis (thrush). Consider prescribing an anti-candidiasis pessary/cream on the PRN side of the drug chart.
• Warn women taking the oral contraceptive pill that antibiotics (and other drugs affecting liver metabolism) reduce its efficacy.
• Consider giving at least 24 hours IV treatment if the patient is very unwell.
• Check the *BNF* and local guidelines for the most current treatment of different infections.
• Gentamicin, netilmicin and vancomycin need regular peak and trough levels (see the *BNF* or phone pharmacology).

Standard treatments for common infections include
Chest infection
Oral amoxicillin (erythromycin if penicillin allergic)
Second choice: erythromycin or ciprofloxacin
You do not need to give erythromycin *and* amoxicillin unless there is consolidation

Severe infection or hospital acquired infection
IV cephalosporin, for example cefuroxime

Aspiration pneumonia
Amoxicillin and metronidazole

UTI
Oral trimethoprim *or* cephalosporin *or* ciprofloxacin

Cellulitis
Flucloxacillin and amoxicillin

Septicaemia
IV cefuroxime and gentamicin (see hospital policy)

Anticoagulation

House Officers are often required to anticoagulate patients following unstable angina, heart attacks, DVTs and PEs. Ask your colleagues for local protocols. These generally involve giving heparin and warfarin together, then stopping the heparin once the INR is high enough (i.e. when the warfarin begins to work).
1 Check that the patient has no bleeding disorder. Do FBC, INR and APTT.

2 If using unfractionated intravenous heparin:

Start the patient on a heparin pump (usually 25 000 units in 50 ml of normal saline, run at 2.8 ml/hour (1400 units/hour). Check the APTT at least once a day and adjust the heparin according to a sliding scale (see the *BNF*). Ideally, the APTT should hover around 1.5–2.5. The heparin should be stopped if the APTT is more than 7.

If using low molecular weight heparin:

Prescribe daily subcutaneous low molecular weight heparin. Each hospital has its own preferred brand; check with your formulary and weight-adjust the dose as per *BNF* guidelines. Dosing regime will vary with brand and indication. APTT need not be checked.

3 Start the patient simultaneously on warfarin. The standard protocol is:

• Give 10 mg of warfarin on the first day, 5 mg on the second and third, then adjust according to the INR. This protocol may need to be modified for the elderly, frail, those with liver disease and on liver-stimulating drugs. Check with your senior.

• You need to check the INR daily from the first dose. Reduce the warfarin dose if the INR rises too quickly or too high (for example, above 5).

• The INR needs to be checked:

Every day for 1 week

Every week for 3 weeks

Every month for 3 months

Every 8 weeks after that

Always inform the GP in the discharge summary that the patient has been started on warfarin and that the INR will need to be checked.

• You are usually aiming for an INR of 2–3 (but this varies depending on the condition; check the *BNF*).

• Clearly explain the potential side effects of warfarin to the patient and that they must inform their GP and any other health professional that they are taking warfarin. It is also advisable to tell the patient to keep tablets well hidden from small children. Advise patients to let their pharmacist know that they are taking warfarin before buying over-the-counter medications.

• If the INR or APTT are too high, simply stop the warfarin and/or heparin. If the INR is greater than 10, or the patient is bleeding, give 4 units of FFP and recheck the clotting. A small dose (1–2 mg) of vitamin K will reverse the clotting in a few hours. Beware of giving higher doses as this prevents further anticoagulation for weeks. Always consult with a haematologist and colleagues if a patient is in danger of bleeding. Beware of anaphylaxis (be prepared to treat with O_2 and adrenaline, see p. 87). FFP can also be given stat to decrease a bleeding tendency. Heparin can be reversed with protamine sulphate. Use 1 mg protamine sulphate/100 iu of heparin, to a maximum of 50 mg. This should work within half an hour.

Anti-emetics (see Nausea and vomiting p. 76)

Digoxin

Digoxin is a commonly used drug to slow down the ventricular rate in atrial fibrillation. It is potentially dangerous with many side effects, such as fatigue, confusion, N&V, anorexia, diarrhoea and arrhythmias. Digoxin also interacts with many drugs (see the *BNF*). In particular, beware of drugs which lower K (for example, diuretics), as hypokalaemia predisposes to digoxin toxicity.

How to digitalize (discuss with your senior first)

1 In the non-acute situation:
   • Give the patient 125–250 µg (micrograms) of digoxin twice daily for 1 week. No loading dose is required.
   • Reduce dose to once daily for maintenance. Digoxin maintenance dosage varies according to age, weight and renal function. In general:
   Normal dose 125–375 µg.
   In the elderly 62.5–125 µg.
   If renal impairment, discuss with pharmacologist.
   • If the patient experiences side effects, measure digoxin levels for toxicity. Digoxin-specific antibodies are now available as an antidote to digoxin poisoning.

2 In the acute situation (for more rapid control of the ventricular rate):
   • Give 500 µg of digoxin 8-hourly until the rate is controlled (usually takes 3–4 doses), then give the maintenance dose (see above), *or*
   • Give 500 µg IV and 500 µg orally at the same time, then continue with maintenance doses. This method is faster.

Night sedation (see Insomnia p. 72)

Be wary of giving night sedation without making sure that the patient does not need further medical attention or better day management.

Therapeutic drug levels

House Officers are sometimes required to check the blood levels of several commonly used drugs (Table 9.2). This involves liaising with the nurse giving the drug so that you can take blood for levels at the appropriate times (for example, at peak and trough dosage times). Ask the biochemistry technicians which tube to use (usually a biochemistry tube).

Steroids (see The steroid patient, p. 115)

Miscellaneous tips

• Metronidazole can be given easily and cheaply as a suppository. This is particularly useful after an appendicectomy, if the patient does not need a drip.
• Metronidazole bags for IV use can be requested from pharmacy. You can ask the pharmacist to add cefuroxime so that you don't have to do IV drug rounds for either (the nurses put them up). Store the bags in the fridge and watch the use-by date.
• If a drug risks causing anaphylaxis (for example, phytomenadione), ensure that you have adrenaline ready and a resuscitation trolley available. *Do not leave the ward for about 5 minutes after giving these drugs.*
• Any drug which is protein-based can cause anaphylaxis.
• Always consider prescribing laxatives prophylactically with opiate analgesia.
• Steroid conversion (also see p. 115):
   0.75 mg dexamethasone = 5 mg prednisolone = 20 mg hydrocortisone = 25 mg cortisone.

Table 9.2 Therapeutic drug levels and sampling times.

Drug	Sampling time	Therapeutic range
Amiodarone	Any time when blood levels are stable (after 1 month)	0.6–2.5 mg/l
Carbamazepine	Peak 3 hours after dose	Single therapy: 8–12 mg/l Multiple therapy: 4–8 mg/l
Digoxin	At least 6 h after dose Check C&E and Ca, as toxicity is potentiated if Ca is high or K is low	0.8–2 μg/l
Gentamicin and tobramicin	Peak 1 hour after dose Trough (just before new dose)	Peak 5–10 mg/l Trough <2 mg/l
Lithium	12 hours after dose	0.4–1.0 mmol/l
Phenytoin	IV peak 2–4 hours after dose Oral peak 3–9 hours after dose	10–20 mg/l
Sodium valproate	Plasma levels are not a good guide to efficacy	
Vancomycin	Peak 1 hour after dose Trough Also check C&E for renal toxicity	25–40 mg/l 1–3 mg/l

• Consider pre-emptive prescribing (i.e. prescribing certain drugs on the PRN side of the chart for all patients without contraindications) to prevent nurses bleeping you and your colleagues: paracetamol, temazepam (see above), laxatives.

Chapter 10: **Handle with care**

Some patients require special attention as they are especially vulnerable due to physical or mental frailty, and stigma.

Alcoholism

Many more of your patients will be addicted to alcohol than you realize. To assess alcoholism, do the CAGE questionnaire,* which is remarkably reliable for picking up alcoholism:

1 Have you ever felt you should C UT down on drinking?
2 Have people made you A NGRY by asking about your alcohol intake?
3 Have you ever felt G UILTY about your drinking?
4 Do you ever drink first thing in the morning (or take an E YE OPENER)?

Answering 'yes' to two or more of the above questions gives the patient an 80% chance of having an alcohol problem.

• Ask the patient for a typical day, with the amount and type of alcohol taken at each time.
• Tactfully ask relatives or friends about the patient if you suspect denial of alcoholism.
• Do an MCV (with FBC) and GGT. Both rise with prolonged use of alcohol, and take approximately 2–3 months to

---

* Mayfield D., McLeod G., Hall P. (1974) The CAGE questionnaire: validation of a new alcoholism screening instrument. *American Journal of Psychiatry* 131, 1121–1123.

---

return to normal following abstention. If these are raised, discuss the findings with the patient and your colleagues regarding further treatment.

• Women should not drink more than 21 units/week; men 28 units/week. One unit contains 8 g of alcohol. Drinks containing 1 unit of alcohol include a half pint of beer, a small glass of red or white wine, a single bar serving of spirits or sherry or fortified wine.
• Consider a nutritional screen and vitamin supplements (especially the B, D and K groups).

Alcohol withdrawal

Some patients will be admitted specifically to withdraw from alcohol; others will have their alcoholism unmasked in hospital. Always consider alcohol (and nicotine) withdrawal if your patient suddenly becomes unexpectedly ill or agitated.

• Ask your senior for local protocols.
• Watch for hypotension, dehydration, hypoglycaemia and electrolyte imbalance. Ensure 4-hourly observation and regular U&E, glucose, FBC.
• Prescribe clomethiazole as shown in Table 10.1. Do not treat with clomethiazole for more than 9 days. *Note that lorazepam is rapidly superseding the use of clomethiazole in some centres. It is cheaper and more effective. Ask your senior for their preference.*
• Consider IV clomethiazole if the patient is vomiting. A 0.8% infusion of

Table 10.1 Prescribing clomethiazole. Do not treat with clomethiazole for more than 9 days.

Day	Number of clomethiazole tablets	Tablet timing
Day 1	2–4	6 hourly
Day 2	2–3	6 hourly
Day 3	1–2	9 hourly
Days 4–9	Gradually decrease dose	

clomethiazole at 3–7.5 ml (24–60 mg)/minute, reducing to 0.5–1 ml (4–8 mg)/minute, should keep the patient lightly sedated. Consult with your senior before administering IV clomethiazole. A resuscitation trolley must be available and frequent observations performed, as the patient may become too deeply sedated.

• Be careful with clomethiazole. Patients should not drive for 48 hours after taking the last dose. Sedation may mask hepatic coma. Avoid prolonged use and abrupt withdrawal. Dependence becomes a problem after about 9 days.

• Randomized controlled trials suggest that patients are likely to do better if they are initially detoxified in hospital, as opposed to being managed solely in the community.*

Children

You may work with children as a surgical House Officer, although you are not expected to provide full paediatric care. These tips may help:

• Remove your white coat before working with children. It helps to avoid doctor phobia and unnecessary formality.

• For children under 14, get consent from parents/guardians while they are on the ward, or you will have to call them in from home.

• Minors between 14 and 16 can legally sign for themselves, but it is usually a good idea to get parental or guardian consent.

• Ask the anaesthetist to insert cannulae when the child is asleep for theatre, to minimize needle trauma and phobia.

• Use paediatric blood bottles (available on paediatric wards and in the paediatric room in casualty) to minimize blood letting.

• Use local anaesthetic cream before inserting cannulae and taking blood.

• Be cautious when prescribing IV fluids and drugs—different sized children have very different fluid and drug needs. Consult the *BNF* and colleagues if in doubt.

• If you are desperate for a vein, children under about 10 months have good scalp veins which can be accessed using a blue butterfly.

Depression

People in hospital are often depressed—with good reason. Hospitals can be scary,

* Walsh D.C., Hingson R.W., Merrigan D.M. *et al.* (1991) A randomized trial of treatment options for alcohol-abusing workers. *New England Journal of Medicine* **325**, 775–782.

lonely places even if you are well, let alone facing serious illness and death.

• Be alert to sudden mood changes and negative conversation. Ask patients about their fears. You may be able to help immediately with reassurance or liaisons with social workers, nurses, psychiatrists and medical colleagues.

• Interestingly, many elderly patients suffering from acute conditions such as MI or strokes have been recently bereaved. Your patient may be grieving.

• If your patient seems low, they may be suffering from occult pain, hypoxia, alcohol or drug withdrawal, electrolyte and thyroid imbalances, as well as concerns about employment, home care and other likely worries.

• Alert psychiatrists and colleagues if you think a patient is in danger of attempting suicide (see p. 21).

Elderly patients

Like children, elderly patients can present with non-specific, under-stated symptoms. Elderly patients are often stoical and may hide quite severe pain.

1 Monitor vital signs. Breathe with the patient to exclude quiet tachypnoea. Consider checking rectal temperature.

2 Go through a checklist of systems to make sure you're not missing something serious. In particular, watch for;

• Fractures: old people often don't complain of pain. *Look* at the limbs (especially the hips, legs and wrists) and feel for crepitus.

• Hypoxia: people may present with euphoria. Measure the respiratory rate and do pulse oximetry or blood gases if concerned.

• Fluid overload and electrolyte im-

balance: check IV fluids, electrolytes and slow down or stop fluids if necessary. A basic IV fluid regime for elderly people is:

Normal saline
   500 ml + KCl 20 mM
    Over 6 hours
Normal saline
   500 ml + KCl 20 mM
    Over 6 hours
5% Dextrose
   500 ml + KCl 20 mM
    Over 6 hours
5% Dextrose
   500 ml
    Over 6 hours

and monitor electrolytes daily. Reconsider whether the patient needs IV fluids.

• Hypothermia: consider checking rectal temperature.

• Malnutrition: look for flaky skin, poor gums, unhealed bruises or scratches. Consider a nutritional screen.

• K-wasting with diuretics. Check K and supplement orally if necessary. Be careful not to produce hyperkalaemia. If you send the patient home with K supplements, be sure to notify both the patient and the GP, so K can be monitored.

• Infantilization of elderly patients. Remember that 80% of elderly patients live at home. Only 14% of people over 75 have any form of dementia. Be careful not to treat elderly people like children.

Haemophiliacs

All in all, haemophiliacs get a bad deal. Most adult UK haemophiliacs are Hep

B/C and/or HIV-positive. Haemophilia can be crippling, as members of various royal families can testify. People with haemophilia often have many bad hospital experiences. More than most, this group needs open and honest communication. Because of the high rate of infectivity, you need to take the following precautions.

Taking blood

• Minimize taking blood. Question your colleagues if they have requested frequent routine bloods.

• Phone a haematologist or (ideally) the nearest haemophiliac service. Usually they will take blood for you (ask the haematologist where the nearest service is).

• Use paediatric bottles from the paediatrics ward to minimize the amount of blood needed.

• Never use a vacutainer; its 18 gauge needle is too big. Use the smallest possible needle or blue butterfly on small veins. Knuckle veins can be useful.

• Never use a tourniquet. It causes excessive bruising and occasionally major bleeds from pressure trauma to blood vessels. If you need pressure to find a vein, very gently inflate a blood pressure cuff, but release the pressure as soon as you are in the vein, or you will cause major bruising.

• Never give or prescribe drugs IM.

• Always use standard precautions for taking blood samples. Nearly all UK haemophiliac adults have Hep C, and about two-thirds have HIV.

• Always alert the lab to the haemophiliac status of patient and his or her hepatitis/HIV status.

• Tell patients why you are taking blood and that you are taking care to avoid any unnecessary tests. These patients are often loath to have more blood taken.

For theatre

• Do a full clotting screen (INR, bleeding time, APTT, fibrinogen) preoperatively and a screen for antibodies. Liaise with the haematologist. Any deficiency of factors VIII or IX must be corrected before theatre. If the deficiency is corrected, the patient can be treated like other patients post-operatively, except:

• Factor VIII levels should be tested post-operatively twice per day (factor IX levels once per day). Make sure the first level is taken *before* the patient is bathed and the wound dressed.

• Delay suture removal beyond the usual 10 days, as haemophiliacs are prone to bleeding about this time. Get senior advice.

HIV/AIDS

It goes without saying that these patients need special care. They face both death and stigma. You face potentially dangerous needlestick injuries. Time, care and an honest, open approach are essential.

Taking blood

• It is completely fine to touch HIV/AIDS patients without gloves just about anywhere—just not in a major artery! It is really awful for such patients if health professionals are scared to treat them normally.

• However, do always wear gloves when taking blood. Always have plenty of space for your tray and sharps. Use a nursing trolley if possible and have separate cardboard trays for sharps.

• Don't do things in a hurry. Leave plenty of time for procedures and explanations.

• Label blood samples with high risk stickies (not in front of the patient). These are available from the labs if they are not already on your ward. It is your responsibility if a lab worker contracts HIV from an unlabelled sample.

• Use two specimen bags for high risk samples.

• Always warn theatre staff if a patient has HIV or AIDS.

• Treat oral *Candida* with nystatin lozenges (mild) or ketoconazole/miconazole (see the *BNF*).

• Be aware that HIV/AIDS patients may suffer from depression and may consider suicide. Consider referring to the psychiatrists or social workers. Discuss the patient with the nursing staff—and the patient, of course!

• AIDS patients may suffer from multiple serious medical problems which may require urgent or aggressive therapy. Common problems include: fever, atypical pneumonia, diarrhoea, skin sores, and drug reactions. For reasons that are as yet poorly understood, allergies are much more common in patients with AIDS. If you find yourself looking after an AIDS patient in a general ward, get expert advice from infectious disease staff.

• If necessary reassure non-medical ward staff that they cannot catch HIV from an AIDS patient, so that they don't emit an aura of apprehension that the patient will quickly detect.

HIV testing

Patients need counselling and preparation for HIV tests. Discuss doing HIV tests with seniors; they can advise you on hospital policy. The ward's social worker may be able to help you with this.

• Explain HIV/AIDS. Being HIV-positive is not the same thing as having AIDS. At present 50% of asymptomatic HIV-positive patients get AIDS after 10 years.

• Explain the benefits of the test. If the patient is HIV-positive, you can monitor T cell function, treat infection better, and he or she can practise safe sex and protect his or her partner. 24-hour support is available for people with HIV.

• Explain the problems of the test. Some life insurance companies may discriminate against the HIV-positive person (this is being phased out). A way around this is to get tested anonymously at an STD clinic.

• Arrange with a virologist to have the blood tested as soon as possible (so the patient is not stewing for days).

• Label the sample carefully and take all precautions when taking it.

• Tell the patient at what time the result will be back. If there is any delay, let the patient know and reassure him or her that it is not due to the sample being infected.

Jehovah's Witnesses/ Christian Scientists

• As with any person, you cannot force a Jehovah's Witness or Christian Scientist to accept treatment (for example, a blood transfusion). Make sure they sign a statement acknowledging refusal of treatment. Most hospitals have policy documents and suitable consent or exemption forms. Discuss the case with your seniors.

• In an emergency, you can legally instigate treatment to save someone's life unless it is clear that the patient has given an informed refusal of that treatment which remains in force. Again, get nursing and senior advice and, if necessary, advice from your defence organization.

Pregnant women

• Get senior advice about X-rays in pregancy (see p. 180). Make sure you notify the radiologist that the patient is pregnant—write it clearly on the form and preferably speak to the radiologist yourself.

• Always ask women of child-bearing age the date of their LMP and whether or not they are likely to be pregnant.

• Pregnant women have hyperdynamic, volume-expanded circulations. Their JVPs are usually slightly raised. This is okay, but it also means that they can lose a lot of blood before they exhibit signs of hypovolaemia.

• Most drugs are potentially toxic. Make sure you know the trimester and always get senior or pharmacist advice before prescribing.

• Fetuses are like enormous tumours. They consume folate, iron, Ca and other vitamins that would normally go to the mother. Ensure that pregnant women have adequate nutrition and supplement if necessary.

• Be wary of pregnant women with abdominal pain. Organs such as the appendix get displaced, and inflammation can present in bizarre ways. For example, appendicitis may present as chest pain if it irritates the diaphragm. Always seek senior advice. Consider notifying an obstetrician.

Sickle cell anaemia

Be alert to sickle cell anaemia in any black, Arabic, Indian or Mediterranean patient within the UK with acute pain in the spine, joints, chest or abdomen. Within the UK, all patients of African descent need a sickling test before surgery. Heterozygous patients are only likely to suffer severe symptoms when hypoxic, as may occur during anaesthesia or at high altitudes. However, in homozygous patients, sickling crises are precipitated by hypoxia, infection, cold and other common stressors. Sickling crises can develop with alarming rapidity and can be fatal without prompt treatment. The patient will often know when they are going into crisis.

1 Symptoms of a sickle crisis include severe bone pain, acute abdominal pain, SOB and neurological symptoms such as fits and cranial nerve palsies.

2 Basic management includes prompt **analgesia** (pethidine 100–200 mg IM 2 hourly as required), O_2 therapy, **rehydration** (ensure fluid intake of at least 3 l/day) and **antibiotics** if pyrexial or evidence of infection. Make sure the patient is warm. Seek urgent, expert help especially if they do not improve quickly—these patients can deteriorate within hours! Lung involvement is particularly worrying.

3 Investigations: the patient will need urgent IV access and baseline bloods, cross-match, FBC, reticulocyte count

and film, blood cultures, MSU and chest X-ray. Include ABGs if there is any CXR-shadowing, respiratory symptoms or infection). Measure Hb daily.

4 If the patient needs surgery, seek specialist anaesthetic advice.

The steroid patient

Patients on steroids are vulnerable to infection and other side effects, and may require additional steroid cover while ill. Steroids affect the immune system, fluid balance, carbohydrate, lipid and protein metabolism. Anti-inflammatory steroid equivalent doses are shown in Table 10.2.

Side effects of steroids

Mineralocorticoid
Na and water retention, hypertension
Hypokalaemia

Glucocorticoid
Diabetes
Changes in fat distribution
Changes in protein mobilization: osteoporosis, skin atrophy, striae, muscle wasting, delayed wound healing

Mental changes
These occur in most patients. They vary from subtle changes to frank paranoid psychosis. Warn the patient (and relatives and friends!) that they may become easily irritable or 'difficult' and that they should inform the doctor if this causes problems. Initial euphoria and increased appetite are common

Table 10.2 Anti-inflammatory steroid equivalent doses.

Steroid	Dose (mg)
Dexamethasone and betamethasone	0.75
Methylprednisolone and triamcinolone	4
Prednisolone	5
Hydrocortisone	20

Infection
Candida infection: oesophageal (dysphagia) or vaginal (itching)
Disseminated viral infection: measles, varicella zoster and herpes zoster
Bacterial infection. The inflammatory response is suppressed hence late presentation and rapid systemic spread of infection. Be alert to the 'silent' abdomen, septicaemia and TB

Others
Peptic ulceration: severe dyspepsia is common although the link to ulceration is less well understood
Acne is common
Withdrawal reactions (see below)

Managing ill patients on steroids

Illness (acute stress, especially surgery or infection) increases steroid requirements. Decide if your patient needs additional steroids or not. Prescribe hydrocortisone 25–100 mg tds (or equivalent) in addition to existing steroid dose if required. See p. 195 for surgical steroid cover. Always be aware of 'silent' infections in a patient on high dose steroids (see side effects).

Treating common side effects

1 *Candida* infection. Prescribe nystatin lozenges or miconazole oral gel for oral/oesophageal infection, and clotrimazole (Canesten) cream/vaginal pessaries for vaginal infection. Fluconazole 50 mg PO daily is useful as prophylaxis for high dose steroids.

2 If the patient is known to suffer from cold sores or shingles, tell the patient to start high dose acyclovir at the earliest sign of recurrence.

3 Heartburn. Prescribe ranitidine 150 mg nocte or equivalent.

Withdrawing steroid therapy

The longer the patient has been on steroids, the more gradual the reduction of steroids needs to be. Abrupt withdrawal may cause acute adrenal insufficiency or Addisonian crisis. Therapy for longer than 2 weeks can lead to adrenal suppression.

You can reduce steroids from high doses by 5–10 mg of prednisolone (or equivalent)/week until you reach the equivalent of 10 mg prednisolone/day. Thereafter, reduce by 2.5 mg/week until you reach 5 mg/day. After this, the rate of reduction depends on the preceding length of therapy. If this was greater than 3 months, reduce slowly, e.g. by 1–2 mg/week.

Withdrawal reactions

Addisonian crisis (hypotension, dehydration, hyperkalaemia, hyponatraemia), arthralgia, conjunctivitis, mood change, rhinitis, skin rashes—itchy nodules or acne, weight loss. Morning irritability can be prevented by taking the daily dose bd.

Chapter 11: **Approach to the medical patient**

A major task during medical house jobs is clerking patients. This section provides a practical approach to history and examination of the medical patient, and how to optimize your time in getting to know the patient and in getting a feel for their problems.

In general, with the introduction of shift work, you may find yourself looking after a patient you did not admit and do not know. It is well worth the effort to re-clerk these patients as soon as possible. It takes much less time than you think and will allow you to develop a better relationship with the patient. While your night-shift colleagues are unlikely to miss an obvious sign, it is remarkable how much more information is yielded by a history taken in the light of day.

An approach to history taking comprises two essential parts, which enable management to be tailored to the individual patient and his or her disease:
1 Getting to know the patient (the person and their medical background).
2 Getting to know the disease (the presenting problem).

Getting to know the patient as a person

- Patient ID — age, sex, etc.
- Work.
- Lives with.
- Social support — family, friends, finances.

- Mobility.
- Home help.
- Problems as perceived by the patient: worries, fears.

The medical background

- Past medical history.
- Past surgical history.
- What operations and any anaesthetic complications?
- Allergies, drug history.
- Family history.

Getting to know the disease

Presenting complaints. Identify as clearly as possible the reason for the patient presenting now and think of the possible causes for the symptoms so that you establish an early ranked differential diagnosis. Do not take a history blindly, without this kind of forethought. Be aware of the diagnostic possibilities based on the background and the presenting complaint so that you ask questions that strengthen or refute a specific possibility. At this stage it is useful to stop, think and construct a ranked differential diagnosis before the next phase of the history taking.

The present history. This is what the patient tells you about their present illness. Listen carefully and ask clarifying questions. Attempt to live the patient's life from the onset of the symptoms so that you become aware of important details that will refine your differential diagnosis. Next, try to refine your differential diagnosis and identify those features of the most likely diseases that have emerged thus far. Ask about these features now — *the specific directed enquiry*, and write down your differential diagnosis and problem list before the examination.

The systematic (or functional) enquiry. This is usually the least useful part of the history. While it provides a convenient list of symptoms, it encourages thoughtless history taking that overworked junior doctors don't need! It should therefore be left until last but not omitted. For the detailed list of symptoms see Fig. 11.1.

The examination

The same general examination for all patients should be followed by a directed systemic examination, based on the diagnostic possibilities elicited in your history. For example, you would make a careful check for signs of infective endocarditis in a patient with a history of valvular heart disease and recent decrease in exercise tolerance. Note the important negative findings, for example, no splinter haemorrhages, no vasculitic skin lesions, no splenomegaly. Fully document your findings.

We provide an outline of the general and systematic examination of the medical patient on p. 120. While it is structured in the order for 'routine' examination, few patients are 'routine', and you should examine some systems in more detail according to your differential diagnosis.

Summing up

At the end of your history and examination, it is a good idea to sum-up for presenting on ward rounds.

1 Patient ID and salient medical background. (Mention only that which is pertinent to the present problem.)

2 Presenting complaint.

3 Current problems — medical, pharmacological, social.

4 Investigations.

5 Plan for discharge — how the team is going about solving the patient's problems and the likely time of discharge from hospital.

History and examination

Figures 11.1 and 11.2 provide an outline of the above approach to history and examination. Re-type and photocopy if you want.

Clinical stalemate

Your patient sits in bed day after day, and no progress is made. What do you do?

1 Decide if the patient is sick or not, and getting better or getting sicker day by day. Sometimes you should let well alone.

2 If the patient is ill or getting worse, then rapidly identify the main problems and make a management plan, for example is the renal function, mental state or pulmonary function deteriorating?

3 Having addressed obvious problems, review the case. It can be helpful to 're-clerk' the patient, especially as this clerking will have the benefit of

History

Getting to know the patient as a person

Patient ID—age, sex, etc.

Work .... Mobility ....

Lives with .... Home help ....

Social support— Problems as perceived by the patient,

family, friends .... worries, fears ....

Finances ....

The medical background

Past medical history

1 CVS–IHD, rheumatic fever, hypertension, other

2 RS–asthma, smoker, TB, exposure to irritants

3 Diabetes, thyroid disease, other medical illnesses

Past surgical history

What operations

Any anaesthetic complications

Drug history and allergies

Current medication

Relevant past medication

Allergies

Family history

Hobbies and pets

Getting to know the disease

Presenting complaint/s

(STOP–THINK–CONSTRUCT A RANKED DIFFERENTIAL DIAGNOSIS)

The present history and the specific directed enquiry

(What the patient tells you about their illness and directed questions to define the differential.)

Systematic (or functional) enquiry

1 General–loss of appetite, loss of weight, fever, night sweats, any lumps, itch and rashes.
2 CVS/RS–chest pain, dyspnoea, orthopnoea, PND, cough, haemoptysis, sputum, ankle oedema, intermittent claudication.
3 GIT–dyspepsia, nausea, vomiting, diarrhoea, change in bowel habit, blood or mucus PR.
4 GU–dysuria, frequency, urgency, nocturia, haematuria, polyuria, incontinence.
5 Gynaecology–vaginal discharge, menses, first day of last period (LMP), menarche, menopause, pregnancy.
6 CNS–fits, blackouts, headaches, visual disturbances, sensory disturbances, weakness/paralysis, falls, loss of hearing. Higher mental function.
7 MSK/skin–joint pain/swelling, stiffness.

Refined differential diagnosis

Fig. 11.1 Approach to history taking.

Examination

In order of examination

1. Appearance. Does the patient look ill? General nutrition
2. Temperature

Working up the arm:

3. Hands, nails
4. Pulse
5. Respiratory rate
6. While doing the above, consider evidence of endocrine disease (pituitary, thyroid, Addisons), Paget's; body hair, skin pigmentation, skin lesions
7. BP
8. Eyes–pallor, jaundice
9. Mouth and tongue–cyanosis, smooth or furred tongue, any lesions?
10. Examine the neck–nodes, goitre

CVS examination with patient at 45°:

11. JVP and cartoid pulses
12. Praecordium–inspect, palpate, auscultate
13. Sacral oedema? Ankle oedema?

RS examination with patient at 90°:

14. Chest–inspect, palpate (trachea, expansion), auscultate
15. Breasts and axillary nodes

GIT examination with patient lying flat:

16. Abdomen–inspect, palpate (tenderness, visceromegaly), auscultate (bowel sounds)

Legs:

17. Swelling, pulses

CNS examination:

The detail of this examination will depend on the differential diagnosis. The essentials include:

18. Cranial nerves–pupil responses; fundi; corneal reflexes; 'Open your mouth; stick out your tongue; show me your teeth; shut your eyes tightly; raise your eyebrows; shrug your shoulders'
19. Peripheral nerves and motor function–wasting; sensation (vibration, light touch); tone; power; gait
20. Speech and higher mental functions
21. Do PR and FOB test. Consider PV
22. Dipstick urine and consider microscopy
23. Summarize findings and list your plan for solving the patient's problems:
    - Patient ID and salient medical background
    - Presenting complaint/s ....
    ....
    - Current problem/s ....
    ....
    - Investigations ....
    ....
    - Plan for discharge ....
    ....

Fig. 11.2 Approach to examination.

hindsight, and the use of previous notes, the patient's drug chart, etc.

- Main complaint.
- History of main complaint.
- PMH.
- Drugs, allergies, habits, travel, etc.

4 Repeat a complete examination. Like the history, the examination will benefit from hindsight and recent investigation results. Examine test results critically — are they reliable or spurious? Are they up to date?

5 Formulate now a list of problems, differential diagnoses, and investigations to be requested. You may not come up with blinding new answers immediately, but you will know the case a lot better, and you will avoid the embarrassment of having overlooked key pieces of information in the history, examination and investigations.

6 Now write a summary in the notes of your findings at this stage. If appropriate, use tables for important serial data.

Preparing patients for medical procedures

During your house job you will prepare patients for many different procedures. This section explains what needs to be done and what complications to expect. It is important to realize that while most procedures are routine for you, they are usually frightening for patients. Probably the scariest thing is not knowing what will happen next, so lots of information can make a big difference. A list of patients' common concerns about procedures includes:

1 What does the procedure entail?
2 Why are they having this done?
3 How long will the procedure take?

4 Do they need a general anaesthetic?
5 Will the procedure be painful?
6 What should they do if they have pain or other symptoms after the procedure?
7 When can they eat/drink/drive/talk/have sex?
8 Will they have any scars/permanent after-effects?
9 Who is doing the procedure?

Cardiac catheterization

Preparation

1 Consent (if angioplasty or stenting is planned in addition to diagnostic catheterization, this should be explained. There are variants of the procedure, for example, left and right heart catheters, coronary angiography, electrophysiological studies, depending on the indication. Ask the cardiologists what they intend. If unsure how to consent accurately, ask them for help). Informed consent may only be obtained by the person doing the procedure, although you can make their job easier by explaining the procedure to the patient.

2 Make sure the patient has stopped oral anticoagulants at least 3 days prior to the procedure. In some cases, for instance, when a patient has a metal valve replacement, the patient should be admitted for heparinization, since this can be discontinued a few hours prior to the procedure.

3 Request FBC, platelets, INR, APTT, G&S, U&E and creatinine to check renal function.

4 Secure peripheral venous access.

5 Check all peripheral pulses (this acts as a baseline, since rarely, cardiac catheterization can cause peripheral arterial thromboembolism).

6 If the patient has renal impairment or diabetes, seek senior advice.

Consider telling patient

1 Why they require cardiac catheterization.

2 The procedure will be done under local anaesthetic and sometimes mild sedation, via the blood vessels in the groin (although sometimes a brachial approach is used via the antecubital fossa, particularly where the patient is anticoagulated).

3 The procedure takes place in a special clinic (called the 'cath lab'), under X-ray guidance.

4 The process may be diagnostic (coronary arteriogram, left ventriculogram and sometimes right ventriculogram, which requires an additional, transvenous approach) or therapeutic (angioplasty or stent).

5 Afterwards, the patient will need to lie flat for about 4 to 6 hours.

6 In some centres, routine diagnostic angiography is done as a day case. Check, and let patients know when they are likely to be allowed home.

7 Afterwards, there may be some bruising, and sometimes an ache in the groin, but this should subside.

Complications

1 Bleeding/bruising at groin puncture site.

2 False aneurysm in groin.

3 Stroke, death, MI (risk is <1/100, but varies with the details of the procedure and baseline characteristics of the patient—ask the cardiologists what risk you should quote for the procedure intended).

Following the procedure

1 Patients are usually taken over by cardiologists following therapeutic cardiac catheterization of a general medical inpatient.

2 Patients must lie flat for several hours.

3 Check groin wound is clean, and there is no evidence of false aneurysm before discharge.

Elective DC cardioversion

Preparation

1 ECG (check that patient is still in atrial fibrillation, and that there are no ventricular abnormalities, for example frequent ectopy).

2 INR (check that INR is currently >2.0, and has been for the last month).

3 U&E: check that serum potassium >3.5 mmol/l, and that other electrolytes are in the normal range.

4 Patient has been NBM for 4 hours prior to attempted cardioversion.

5 If patient is taking digoxin, exclude symptoms of digoxin toxicity (nausea, diarrhoea, visual disturbance, confusion).

6 Peripheral venous access.

7 If the patient has renal impairment, seek senior advice.

8 Inform the anaesthetist and the staff who are required for the procedure. In some centres, the procedure is carried out in theatre recovery or in the induction room, in which case the theatre manager needs to be informed. In other places, it is done on the cardiac day ward, in which case the ward staff should be informed.

9 Obtain informed consent (ask a

senior if you are unsure what risks to quote for a particular patient).

10 Ensure that the skin overlying the right sternal border and the cardiac apex is shaved.

Consider telling the patient

1 Why they require DC cardioversion.

2 It is done under a brief general anaesthetic.

3 What the procedure involves (see below under practical procedures).

4 There is no guarantee that it will cause reversion to sinus rhythm, but that successful cardioversion should bring symptomatic benefit. (The probability of success is highly variable. In young people with no structural heart disease and fairly recent onset, the chances of success are very high; in older people with structural abnormalities and chronic AF, the chances are slim.)

5 Procedure is usually a day case. The patient can go home once the anaesthetic has worn off, but should be taken home by somebody else, and should not drive or operate machinery for the rest of the day.

Complications

1 Small risk of major complication (thromboembolism, life-threatening arrhythmias, aspiration).

2 Skin burns where pads were applied.

Following the procedure

1 Check ECG.

2 Inform patient that the procedure was successful/unsuccessful. If successful, warn patient that effects may not be sustained indefinitely, and that AF may re-occur.

3 Continue medications and arrange outpatient clinic appointment. You may need to check these arrangements with a senior colleague.

4 Wait for 2–3 hours before discharging. Ensure that patients do not go home on their own, and that there is somebody at home to supervise them for the rest of the day.

Upper gastrointestinal endoscopy

Preparation

1 Consent.

2 NBM for 4 hours. If you suspect gastric outlet obstruction, allow only water for 8 hours and NBM for 4 hours.

3 FBC and INR (in case of biopsy).

4 Insert cannula (usually 21 G, although 23 G sometimes suffices) in the arm that will make endoscopic manoeuvring easiest (usually the right arm).

5 Barium can block the suction channel of the endoscope, so delay for 24 hours following upper GI barium studies.

Consider telling the patient

1 What endoscopy is and why they are having it.

2 That the procedure takes about 5–10 minutes, although it may seem longer.

3 During the procedure, they will be given IV sedation, but not a general anaesthetic, to make them drowsy. They shouldn't drive until the following day. Also, their throat will be sprayed with local anaesthetic so that they won't feel the endoscope too much.

4 An endoscope (tube) the thickness of a little finger is passed into the food pipe and into the stomach. It is uncomfortable but not painful.

5 The doctor might take a tiny sample of the inside of the gullet or stomach to examine under a microscope. This is painless.

6 The patient can eat and drink after the local anaesthetic has worn off, which should take about half an hour. They might have a sore throat, which should get better within 1–2 days.

Complications

1 Transient sore throat and possible numbness.

2 Rarely oesophageal perforation (<1 in 1000).

3 Mild bleeding (and rarely haemorrhage) following a biopsy.

Colonoscopy

Preparation

1 Consent.

2 Low residue diet for 36 hours and fluids only for 12 hours before the procedure.

3 Two Picolax sachets (sodium picosulphate and magnesium citrate) or equivalent 24 hours before the procedure. Use one sachet for frail, elderly patients. Do not give to patients with inflamed colonic mucosa (UC, Crohn's, etc.).

Consider telling the patient

1 What colonoscopy is (a way of looking directly at the bowel) and why they are having it.

2 Warn that Picolax causes explosive diarrhoea. They need to drink plenty of clear fluids to maintain hydration (2–3 litres/day: three to four jugs of squash).

3 IV sedation is given that will make them drowsy, but it is not a general anaesthetic (usually).

4 A flexible tube is passed into their back passage.

5 The whole thing takes about 20–30 minutes, and the patient can go home accompanied as soon as the sedation has worn off—usually in about 2 hours. They should not drive until the following day.

Complications

1 Mild abdominal discomfort during and after the procedure is common due to a small amount of gas that is pumped in to aid vision through the colonoscope during the procedure.

2 Incomplete examination, requiring a second examination or barium enema, occurs in about 10% of cases.

3 Perforation occurs about 1 in 500, more commonly in acute colitis or extensive diverticulosis. If this unlikely event happens, the person usually will need to have their bowel repaired under a general anaesthetic.

4 Serious haemorrhage post-biopsy or polypectomy is rare.

Flexible sigmoidoscopy

Preparation

Two phosphate enemas.

Explanation as for colonoscopy except sedation is not usually required.

Liver biopsy

Preparation

1 Consent.
2 Bloods: FBC—Hb and platelets, INR and APTT, liver biochemistry and G&S.
3 Abdominal US advisable to check anatomy (ask the person performing the procedure).
4 Mild pre-med, such as pethidine (50 mg) and prochlorperazine (12.5 mg). Temazepam (10 mg) can also be given if the patient is not at risk of hepatic failure or jaundiced.
5 IV access with at least a green cannula.

Consider telling the patient

1 What a liver biopsy is and why they need one.
2 The procedure is performed on the ward or in an operating theatre. The biopsy itself is very quick (a few seconds) but the whole procedure might take up to 30 minutes—and may seem longer than this. They will have to stay in hospital overnight.
3 The procedure does not usually involve heavy sedation or a general anaesthetic.
4 The site of the biopsy is on the patient's right side, between the 8th and 10th ribs. The patient will need to help by holding their breath during the biopsy.

Complications

1 Shoulder tip or local abdominal pain for a few hours (up to 2 days) is common but relieved by paracetamol 1 g 4–6-hourly.
2 Bleeding possibly requiring transfusion (about 1 in 50).
3 Infection, abscess, pneumothorax (rarely requiring drainage) and biliary peritonitis are uncommon (<1 : 100).

Following the procedure

1 The patient should lie on their right side for at least 2 hours and remain in bed (absolute bedrest) overnight.
2 Observations: BP and pulse every 15 minutes for 1 hour, then every 30 minutes for 2 hours, then hourly for 6 hours. Ask to be informed if the BP falls (>15 mmHg) or if the pulse starts rising (>15 bpm).
3 Ensure that an IV line is secure and that analgesia is written up (ask the operator which they prefer).
4 Check the patient 4 and 8 hours following the biopsy for pain and vital signs.

Pacemaker insertion

Preparation

1 Informed consent.
2 FBC and INR.

Consider telling the patient

1 What a pacemaker is and why he or she needs one.
2 A very small wire is threaded via a large vein (the subclavian) into one of the chambers of the heart under X-ray screening. The wire is gently inserted into the wall of the heart. The other end of the wire is connected to a machine called a pacemaker that generates heart beats, which is placed into a small pocket fashioned in the fatty tissues of the

chest. Its battery will not run out! The pacemaker causes a small lump under the skin on the upper thorax, but nowadays the generators are so small these are hardly noticeable.

3 The procedure is performed under local anaesthetic, sometimes with mild sedation.

4 The procedure is mostly painless. It takes 30–60 minutes.

5 In future, the patient will need to carry a card that says they are fitted with a permanent pacemaker, in case they ever need emergency treatment. A Medicalert bracelet is recommended.

6 Caution in pregnancy, as X-ray screening is used during the procedure.

Complications

1 As for central line placement—pneumothorax, bleeding.

2 Dislodgement of the wire leading to pacing failure. Electrical faults are uncommon.

Following the procedure

1 The patient will need a CXR to check lead placement and to exclude pneumothorax.

2 A pacemaker check ECG to make sure the pacemaker is capturing correctly.

Renal biopsy

Preparation

1 Consent.

2 Bloods: FBC—Hb and platelets, INR, G&S.

3 Abdominal US is essential to check that two kidneys are present.

4 Mild pre-med, such as pethidine (50 mg IM) and prochlorperazine (12.5 mg IM).

5 IV access with at least a green cannula.

Consider telling the patient

1 What a renal biopsy is and why they need one.

2 The procedure is usually done in theatre and takes a few minutes. Sedation is usually required (but not a general anaesthetic).

3 The biopsy is taken through the left or right flank. The patient will need to hold their breath briefly during the biopsy.

4 The patient should drink a lot of fluids after the biopsy, to flush the kidneys and avoid renal colic.

Complications

1 Local pain (prescribe analgesia) and mild haematuria are common.

2 Haemorrhage requiring transfusion is less common (about 1 in 30–60). Surgical intervention for massive haemorrhage is rare.

3 Renal colic from clots may occur.

Following the procedure

1 Patient should lie on the side of the biopsy for at least 2 hours and remain in bed (absolute bedrest) overnight.

2 Observation: BP and pulse every 15 minutes for 1 hour, then every 30 minutes for 2 hours, then hourly for 6 hours. Ask to be informed if the BP falls (>15 mmHg) or if the pulse starts rising (>15 bpm).

3 Check for gross haematuria.

4 Ensure IV access is OK and that good analgesia is written up.

5 Check on the patient 4 and 8 hours following the biopsy for pain, unstable vital signs and gross haematuria or bleeding.

Specialist referrals and investigating the medical case

Most consultants have their own pet investigations. Be guided by ward protocols, but ask someone if you do not understand the rationale for a particular investigation. Protocols often become outdated and nobody takes the time to inform the House Officer.

If a patient is unwell enough to be admitted, you should have the following results to hand:

1 Weight.
2 T.
3 BP.
4 Urine dipstick.
5 FBC and ESR.
6 Biochemistry — at least U&E.

When indicated:

7 CXR.
8 ECG.

Below, we provide a list of further investigations to anticipate, listed under system headings for commonly encountered pathologies. In addition, these are a useful checklist when making specialist referrals. You will greatly impress the admitting consultant if you have useful results to hand. If in doubt, bleep their House Officer to discover which investigations are flavour of the month.

Cardiology

Essential investigations before referral to a cardiologist include ECG and rhythm strip and CXR. In specific situations, see below.

Suspected acute MI

1 Serial ECGs (at least every hour if equivocal and then for three consecutive days).
2 Serial serum cardiac enzymes (some hospitals now offer CK-MB assay which, when taken about 12 hours after the onset of pain, offers a more specific and sensitive marker of MI).
3 If within 6 hours of onset of chest pain, check lipid profile (levels are unreliable after this).

IHD

1 ECG (preferably both during an episode of chest pain and when pain free).
2 Serum cholesterol and triglycerides.
3 Formal blood sugar (ward test is not good enough).

Heart failure (recent onset)

1 ECHO: urgent if there are murmurs of aortic valve disease or you suspect SBE (consider transoesophageal ECHO if local expertise available) or pericardial disease.

Hypertension

1 Cholesterol and triglycerides.
2 MSU for MC&S if blood or protein on urinary dipstick.
3 Ensure there is a recent record of an ECG, CXR and serum biochemistry.
4 US of the kidneys if symptoms are suggestive of clinical renal disease (history of nephritis, renal problems in

childhood, family history of renal disease) or sudden onset or poorly controlled BP.

5 Fundoscopic examination

Infective endocarditis

1 Blood cultures; at least three sets.
2 CRP, C&E and LFT
3 Rh factor.
4 Urine dipstick and microscopy.
5 Blood film, serum haptoglobins and urinary haemosiderin.
6 Consider transoesophageal ECHO.
7 Document peripheral stigmata of infective endocarditis.

Endocrinology

Except for DM, endocrine disorders are rare. Special tests are required according to the differential diagnosis before referral.

Diabetes mellitus

1 Flow chart the patients blood glucose readings and glycosylated Hb (HbA1c) if available.
2 Renal function.
 • Flow chart of creatinine levels.
 • 24-hour urine collection for creatinine clearance and protein.
3 Careful fundoscopy and ophthalmology referral.
4 Peripheral nerve examination.
5 Cholesterol and triglycerides.
6 ECG—have old ECGs to compare.
7 Arrange follow-up in diabetic clinic, arrange diabetic dietary advice by dietician, and involve the diabetic specialist nurse if available.

Investigation of Cushing's

Consult a specialized lab for advice. Different labs prefer different tests.

Standard tests done in most labs include those listed below.

1 10 pm (not necessary to do it at midnight) and 9 am cortisol levels. The night level is usually lower than the morning level, but this diurnal cycle is lost in Cushing's.
2 Shortened low-dose dexamethasone suppression test: 1 mg dexamethasone PO at 11 pm and measure the cortisol level in the morning around 9 am. In Cushing's, the cortisol levels are not suppressed, whereas in pseudo-Cushing's (for example, depression, severe obesity and alcoholism), the cortisol level is suppressed.
3 High dose dexamethasone suppression test: 0.5 mg dexamethasone 6-hourly for 48 hours. Next, measure the morning cortisol level at 24 and 48 hours. This suppresses cortisol levels in pituitary-dependent Cushing's disease, while it does not suppress cortisol levels in adrenal adenomas and ectopic ACTH.
4 Measure urinary-free cortisols (24-hour urine collections).
Note: the best evidence of Cushing's syndrome is the demonstration of loss of diurnal rhythm of cortisol secretion.

Investigations for phaeochromocytoma

Consult a specialized lab for advice. Different labs prefer different tests.

Standard tests done in most labs include those listed below.

1 Three 24-hour urine collections for catecholamines (adrenaline, noradrena-

line metabolites (HMMA/VMA) or total metadrenalines). Requires a special urine bottle. Tell the patient to avoid vanilla, bananas and aspirin.

2 Consider CT or MRI scan of chest and abdomen (phaeo's can arise anywhere along the sympathetic chain), and/or special isotope (MIBG) scan, if the urine test is positive.

Thyroid disease

1 Hypothyroidism: raised TSH, low T_4.

2 Secondary hypothyroidism (rare): low T_4 and T_3 but TSH is not raised; look for pituitary failure.

3 Hyperthyroidism: suppressed TSH and raised T_4 or T_3. In 10% of patients with hyperthyroidism, only the T_3 is raised.

Gastroenterology

Always do a PR before referring to a gastroenterologist.

Gastroenterologists often request some unusual tests. Investigate according to the differential diagnosis.

Upper GI symptoms

1 Faecal occult bloods (×3).
2 Barium meal or gastroscopy.
3 FBC.

GI bleeds (see pp. 63–65)

1 Cross-match.
2 Hb, platelets and clotting studies.
3 Check LFTs, U&E.
4 Endoscopy.
5 Consider surgical consultation.

Chronic diarrhoea

1 Warm stool for MC&S including ova, cysts and parasites (×3), *Clostridium difficile* toxin and culture.
2 FBC (MCV).
3 LFTs (albumin).
4 Ca and phosphate.

Chronic lower GIT symptoms

1 Faecal occult bloods (×3).
2 FBC and MCV.
3 Flexible sigmoidoscopy.
4 Consider barium enema or colonoscopy, depending on local expertise.
5 Consider a small bowel meal.
6 Consider other sources (for example, GU tract) for symptoms.

Ascites of unknown origin

1 History of alcohol consumption.
2 Bloods for LFTs, hepatitis serology. Consider checking anti-mitochondrial antibodies (for primary biliary cirrhosis) and anti-smooth muscle cell antibodies (for chronic active hepatitis).
3 Aspirate the ascites (see p. 169). Re-examine following aspiration, especially the female pelvic organs. A PV is essential if the cause of ascites is unclear.
4 US the abdomen and pelvis (consider aspiration under US guidance if there is a small or loculated collection). US is most useful after aspiration. Specific points on US: Is the portal vein patent? Size and texture of liver and spleen? Porta hepatis nodes?
5 Consider a CT scan.
6 Consider a barium swallow or endoscopy for varices.

7 Consider peritoneoscopy—may be dependent on local expertise.

8 Consider a laparotomy.

Liver disease

1 INR, platelets, bleeding time.

2 Liver biochemistry.

3 Urine for bilirubin and urobilinogen.

4 Hepatitis screen—B and C (A if acute).

5 Iron/TIBC, caeruloplasmin, alpha-fetoprotein.

6 US abdomen.

7 Stool chart.

8 Consider liver biopsy.

9 Consider random alcohol level on this or next admission. MCV and GGT.

Haematology

Essential investigations before referral include FBC, differential, film and ESR.

Suspected DIC

1 FDPs.

2 INR and APTT.

3 LFTs.

4 Urine dipstick and microscopy.

5 Blood cultures.

(DIC is not an end diagnosis—you must find the cause.)

Anaemia (see p. 40)

1 Reticulocyte count ± sickle cell status.

2 Serum bilirubin, LDH (a marker of haemolysis), serum haptoglobins.

3 Iron studies, vitamin B_{12}, serum and red cell folate.

4 CRP, ESR.

5 Consider Hb electrophoresis.

6 Consider bone marrow biopsy.

Suspected paraprotein/myeloma

1 ESR and viscosity.

2 Serum and urine electrophoresis, urine collection for light chains (15% of patients have urinary light chains only).

3 Skeletal survey.

4 Bone marrow biopsy.

Neurology

A thorough history and examination are by far the most important things to do before referral.

Meningism

1 Do LP (see p. 166) if there are no signs of raised ICP (rising BP, papilloedema, depressed LOC). If possible, it is prudent to perform a CT prior to performing LP, to rule out compression of intracranial structures.

• LP pressure.

• MC&S, cell count, xanthochromia.

• Consider Indian ink stains for *Cryptococcus*, ZN for AFBs, viral PCR.

• Glucose.

• Protein.

2 Consider serology for *Cryptococcus*, syphilis and viral causes of meningitis.

3 Consider CT scan head. If suspicious of raised ICP, do CT scan first.

Unexplained coma

Before referral you should:

1 Ensure that the patient's ABC are adequate.

2 Obtain a history from relatives, friends and GP, especially regarding possible drug overdose or recent travel abroad.

3 Do a secondary neurological examina-

tion for clues. The neurological exam would initially have been restricted to the Glasgow Coma Scale and hard localizing signs.

4 Have the following results clearly documented (if available):
• Blood glucose stick that was done immediately on admission.
• FBC, U&E, Ca, phosphate, blood glucose.
• Liver biochemistry.
• Urine dipstick and MC&S.
• ABGs and toxicology screen.

5 Arrange an urgent CT scan head ± LP.
6 Send a serum sample for storage (serology).

Note: MRI scans are becoming a common investigation for neurology patients.

Renal medicine

Renal physicians rely heavily on biochemistry to manage their patients, so have a flow chart of the patient's U&E and creatinine results. Get their help *early* if a patient's renal function is deteriorating.

Renal failure/nephrotics/nephritics

1 BP.
2 Fresh urine for microscopy (do on ward) and send sample for MC&S.
3 Daily weights.
4 Fluid intake/output chart.
5 Serology.
• Virology: CMV, Hep B and C and HIV if candidate for haemodialysis/transplant (remember to counsel the patient).
• Bacteriology: VDRL and atypical serology.

• Immunology: CRP, Igs and serum electrophoresis, complement and autoantibodies; ANA intially, but also consider ANCA, anti-GBM and cryoglobulins.
6 Biochemistry: in addition to renal and hepatic indices request: Ca, total protein, albumin, phosphate.
7 24-hour urine collection—protein and creatinine clearance.
8 Renal US—do early to exclude obstruction, especially if the renal function is deteriorating.
9 Consider renal biopsy.

Renal biopsy (see p. 126)

Recurrent UTIs

1 BP, MSU.
2 Creatinine clearance.
3 Abdominal X-ray to look for calculi. Consider an IVU (looking for structural anomalies).
4 US kidneys (document the size).
5 Consider a micturating cystogram (reflux).
6 PR and proctoscopy.
7 PV and speculum.
8 Consider a urology referral.

Respiratory medicine

Essential investigations before referral to a respiratory physician are CXRs, ECGs and results of lung function tests and ABGs.

Pneumonia

1 CXR.
2 Sputum for MC&S, cytology and AFB.
3 Physiotherapy if bronchopneumonia

or exacerbation of COAD—arrange ASAP. Physiotherapy is not indicated for lobar pneumonia.

4 ABGs are mandatory for any severe respiratory illness.

5 Send a serum sample for storage if you suspect an atypical pneumonia (*Legionella*, *Mycoplasma*, etc).

If you suspect TB

1 Sputum for AFB. (A 5% saline nebulizer will encourage productive coughing if sputum is difficult to obtain.)

2 3× early morning specimens of urine for AFB.

3 Mantoux test (see p. 168).

Obstructive lung disease

Lung function tests pre- and post-bronchodilators.

Respiratory failure

ABGs and acid–base. (Bicarbonate is a useful indicator of chronic CO_2 retention.)

Pleural effusion

1 Send aspirate for:
- Protein, LDH.
- MC&S, AFBs and TB culture.
- Cytology.
- Glucose.

2 Consider pleural biopsy.

3 Consider tuberculin skin test.

Rheumatology

'Look, feel and move' all salient joints. FBC, ESR and CRP. X-rays of relevant joints.

Polyarthritis

1 Urate.

2 Fresh urine for microscopy.

3 X-ray affected joints.

4 CRP.

5 ASOT, serum sample for storage.

6 Latex fixation for Rheumatoid factor.

7 Auto-antibodies screen—ANAs.

8 Consider joint aspiration ± synovial biopsy.

Chapter 12: **Pain**

This section is designed to help you deal with pain control on the general wards. The first section provides a general approach to pain control and summarizes commonly used analgesics, categorized by method of administration (such as inhalational, oral, IM/IV). The boxed section is written by a pain relief specialist. It gives an overview of the crucial and often overlooked aspects of pain control. Finally we provide tables for managing pain according to its severity and underlying clinical conditions.

Pain control

Pain control is critical to good clinical practice, yet it is often poorly managed and poorly understood. Never be afraid to seek senior or specialist advice. Uncontrolled pain is one of the worst things patients can experience. This section gives suggestions for dealing with acute pain most commonly encountered on the wards, many of which also apply to chronic pain.

General

• When first presented with a patient in acute pain, you need to decide whether it is safe to treat the pain symptomatically or whether you should further investigate its cause before masking the symptoms. Do not just treat pain—where possible, find the underlying cause.

• Analgesics are much more effective when used prophylactically. Frequent, mild analgesia may control pain much better than one-off hits of stronger preparations.

• Anticipate common side effects of analgesics, listed in Tables 12.2–12.4. Also be alert to idiosyncratic drug reactions such as rashes and blood dyscrasias.

• You will greatly alleviate acute physical pain by addressing the patient's fear and anxiety. Reassure the patient that the pain can and will be lessened. Next, prescribe an appropriate analgesic (see Tables 12.5 and 12.6).

Specific analgesics

Inhaled drugs (see Table 12.1)

Entonox (50% nitrous oxide, 50% oxygen).

Oral drugs

Paracetamol (see Table 12.2)

Non-steroidal anti-inflammatory drugs (see Table 12.3)

• Aspirin—use of eneteric-coated preparations reduces dyspepsia.

• Naproxen—low incidence of side effects, highly effective for inflammatory pain.

Crucial and often overlooked aspects of pain control

There are two types of pain: acute and chronic. Furthermore, each type of pain has two components: physical (sensory or 'stimulus-dependent') and emotional (Fig. 12.1). In addition, some pain cannot be reduced to physical or emotional components. This is known as 'stimulus-independent' pain. Finally, the relative importance of each component can change, so each patient's pain needs to be assessed daily. Bear in mind that the emotional component is often missed, but may be the most significant contributing factor.

Physical (stimulus-dependent) and stimulus-independent pain

In both acute and chronic pain, the stimulus and the response may not always be

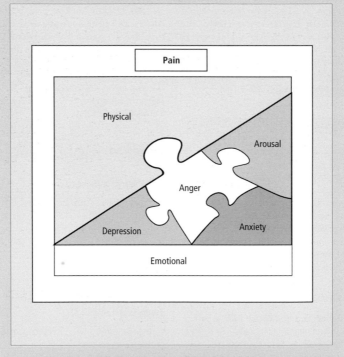

Fig. 12.1 Emotional and physical components of pain.

continued

directly related. There is often background pain independent of the stimulus. Indeed, in chronic pain there may be no relationship between the stimulus and the pain perceived. This 'stimulus-independent' pain is often referred to as neuropathic pain, may be strongly affected by emotion (but not necessarily) and can be extremely difficult to treat. Such pain requires a different approach than stimulus-dependent pain. An example of this is the pain of post-herpetic neuralgia. These patients have altered pain perception: they may be numb to a pinprick but find light touch extremely painful. The most successful treatment for this pain is antidepressants, typifying the enigma of the neuropathic component of pain.

Emotional component of pain

There are four basic mood factors: arousal or awareness, anxiety, unhappiness or depression and anger (Fig. 12.1). The experience of pain is affected—and often heightened—by these different factors.

In *acute pain*, fear and anxiety heightens pain perception. These are usually reduced by treatment with regular pain-killers together with reassurance that pain is to be expected and can be controlled. Occasionally, the emotional response is so intense that it is necessary to use a sedative such as midazolam. For example, arousal (awareness) during procedures is very unpleasant. In endoscopy, opiates are given in combination with sedatives (for example, pethidine and midazolam) thus dealing with both the physical and emotional responses to the stimuli.

In *chronic pain*, the emotional response can include chronic anxiety, depression and anger or frustration, to varying degrees. The clinical significance of these responses needs to be identified and treated. Patients with chronic pain are often angry that the medical profession cannot cure them and may inadvertently vent their frustration on junior staff. Such patients are best referred for treatment at the local pain clinic. Chronic pain patients frequently need help from people very experienced in pain control and in understanding their distress.

• Diclofenac—see naproxen.
• Diflunisal—see naproxen. Longer half-life allows for twice daily doses.
• Ibuprofen—fewer side effects than other NSAIDs though less anti-inflammatory activity.
• Tenoxicam—similar to naproxen. Long half-life allows once daily administration.
• Selective inhibitors of cyclo-oxygenase type-2 (COX-2 inhibitors) are a recent addition to the analgesic armoury. They are as effective as conventional NSAIDs, and it is claimed by the manufacturers that they have fewer GI side effects. They are, however, more expensive.

Contrary to widespread belief, NSAIDs can have GI adverse effects, even when given via non-oral routes.

Opiates (oral)

For pros and cons, see Table 12.4 for IM/IV opiates.

Table 12.1 Entonox (50% nitrous oxide and 50% oxygen).

Pros	Cons
Excellent for one-off or routine painful procedures where the stimulus and response are predictable	Does not work in all patients
	It cannot be used continuously or excessively because it causes bone marrow depression in a dose-dependent manner
Simple, fast and relatively safe	

Note: Never strap the mask in place; you may suffocate the patient. The patient should hold the mask.

Table 12.2 Paracetamol.

Pros	Cons
Few adverse effects	Hepatotoxic in overdose
Useful for mild pain	

Table 12.3 Non-steroidal anti-inflammatory drugs (NSAIDs).

Pros	Cons
Excellent for treating pain associated with inflammation	NSAIDs share many side effects, commonly dyspepsia and nausea
Antipyretic	Occasional GI bleeding/ulceration, diarrhoea
The use of ulcer prophylactic drugs (e.g. H_2 antagonist / proton pump inhibitor) has made the use of NSAIDs safer	Rarely hypersensitivity reactions (angio-oedema, urticaria, bronchospasm); headache; dizziness; vertigo; tinnitus; renal impairment
	Caution in the elderly or if volume depleted (low GFR)
	There is considerable variability in individual patient response to a particular drug
	Can precipitate acute renal failure, especially if there is pre-existing renal impairment

- Codeine—mild to moderate analgesia. High incidence of constipation and drowsiness. N&V are unusual.
- Dihydrocodeine—similar to codeine.
- Morphine (oral)—usually prescribed as slow release preparation. Used for chronic pain in terminally ill patients. High doses are often required as tolerance (tachyphylaxis) develops quite rapidly.

IM/IV opiates

Bolus injection

- This involves slow IV injection over 2–3 minutes.
- Morphine—most commonly used, standard opiate for bad pain (see Table 12.5).
- Pethidine—much weaker analgesic properties than morphine. Most often used as pain prophylaxis for procedures.

Table 12.4 IM/IV opiates.

Pros	Cons
Potent analgesics	Opiates share many side effects, commonly nausea, vomiting, constipation and drowsiness. Respiratory depression and hypotension at higher doses
Excellent for pain relief in the terminally ill Side effects tend to be dose dependent though there is variability between individual patients	
	An anti-emetic is usually required
Naloxone is a highly effective antidote for opiate overdose (hypotension, respiratory depression). Give in incremental doses of 100–200 µg IV every 2 minutes. Beware of overtreating and throwing the patient into severe pain	Addictive

Table 12.5 Recommended analgesics for different levels of pain.

Mild pain
1 Paracetamol 500–1000 mg 4–6-hourly. Max dose in 24 hours is 4 g
2 Aspirin 300–900 mg 4–6-hourly. Max dose in 24 hours is 4 g. Use of enteric coated tablets is recommended to reduce dyspepsia
3 Ibuprofen 400–600 mg 8-hourly. Max dose is 2.4 g daily

Moderate pain
1 Co-dydramol contains paracetamol (500 mg) and dihydrocodeine (10 mg) in each tablet Dose 1–2 tablets 4–6 hourly. Max 8 tablets daily. Remedeine contains paracetamol plus dihydrocodeine in 20 or 30 mg strengths
2 NSAIDs: Diclofenac 75–150 mg PO daily in 2 divided doses; should be taken with food. Dose by IM injection: 75 mg once daily for a max of 2 days. (Max dose 150 mg daily by any route)
3 Codeine 30–60 mg PO/IM 4-hourly. Max dose 240 mg daily. Constipation is common so prescribe a prophylactic laxative (see p. 50)

Severe pain
1 Morphine sulphate 10 mg IM 4-hourly or 2–5 mg IV 4-hourly. (Use 15 mg IM for heavier, well-muscled patients)
2 Diamorphine 5 mg SC/IM 4-hourly or 0.5–2.5 mg/hour IV/SC as an infusion. (Use up to 10 mg IM/SC for heavier, muscular patients)
3 Pethidine 25–100 mg IV/IM/SC repeated after 4 hours. Max dose in 24 hours is 400 mg. Opiates are usually administered with a prophylactic anti-emetic such as prochlorperazine (10 mg PO, 30 minutes before giving the opiate, or 12.5 mg IM)

- Diamorphine—similar analgesic properties to morphine. 5 mg is equivalent to 10 mg of morphine. It is more soluble than morphine, so easier for SC infusions.
- Papaveretum—mixture of morphine, codeine and papaverine. Most commonly used by anaesthetists for perioperative analgesia.

Infusions (SC and PCA)

Morphine and diamorphine are commonly given as continuous infusions,

Table 12.6 Clinical conditions and commonly used analgesics.

Simple headache	Paracetamol
Severe post-op pain	Morphine, pethidine or papaveretum (IM/PO)
Colicky abdominal pain	Hyoscine butylbromide (Buscopan; an antimuscarinic) (PO/IV/IM)
Renal colic	Diclofenac (PO/IM)
Acute MI	Morphine or diamorphine (slow IV injection)
Pleuritic pain	NSAID, e.g. naproxen or diclofenac
Bone pain from metastases	Slow release oral morphine plus NSAIDs
Sciatica	Co-dydramol (mild pain), diclofenac or naproxen (severe pain)
Phantom limb pain	Meprobamate or carbamazepine (consult pain relief clinic)
Diabetic neuropathy	Carbamazepine (consult pain relief clinic)

particularly post-op or in the terminally ill. They can be administered as SC, continuous infusions or can be PCA. Different hospitals use different pumps; ask nursing and medical colleagues how to set up opiate infusions for your patients. Also consult the *BNF* and see p. 102.

Opiate antidote

Naloxone is a highly effective antidote for opiate overdose (small pupils, hypotension, respiratory depression). Give in incremental doses of 100–200 µg IV every 2 minutes. Beware of overtreating, as analgesia may be reversed. Remember that naloxone has a short half-life, so check on the patient later and ask nurses to keep an eye on the patient to ensure they do not slip back into an over-opiated state.

Other

Nerve blockades are rarely given by junior House Officers. The technique for local blockade is described on p. 165. Epidural and spinal blockades are specialist procedures.

TENS (transcutaneous electrical nerve stimulation).

Acupuncture can be very effective for certain types of pain.

Pain control by severity and underlying condition

It is useful to categorize the patient's pain as mild, moderate or severe, and to become familiar with the use of two or three preparations in each category. Our favourite analgesics are listed in Tables 12.5 and 12.6.

Hints

• Many of the compound analgesics contain small doses of codeine or other opiate analgesics. The *BNF* reports that these doses are of little clinical benefit whilst having the potential side effects of opiates. However, some patients swear by them and will only be happy if these are prescribed for their ailment. Common examples are co-proxamol (paracetamol 325 mg plus dextropropoxyphene 32.5 mg) and Co-codamol (paracetamol 500 mg and codeine phosphate 8 mg).

• Ward stocks of compound analgesics may be limited to one or two brands you are not familiar with. Nursing staff will often be able to advise which preparation is the most effective as they will probably have been dispensing the drug to patients for years. Don't be shy to ask for their advice.

Chapter 13: **Practical procedures**

Even those with absolutely no hand–eye coordination can master practical procedures. Most importantly, practice makes perfect. Remember that mistakes are inevitable, so don't be too hard on yourself when you screw up—everyone does. Just be cautious at first and never be afraid to ask for help.

This section is aimed to guide you through most procedures you will encounter as an House Officer. You will no doubt soon develop your own tricks to perfect your performance.

General hints

• Always tell the patient what you are doing and why.
• Never do a procedure unless you have been supervised at least once.
• Order and space make procedures much easier. Before starting a procedure, get everything you need ready on a trolley. Make room for used sharps. Take a sharps bin to where you are working or have a kidney dish ready. Make sure you have enough local anaesthetic, needles and gloves.
• Consider taking the patient to a side room for the procedure, rather than performing it at the bedside which can be embarrassing for the patient and others on the ward.
• A warm, confident approach is most useful even if you are a barrel of nerves inside. It relaxes the patient and in turn will relax you.

• However, never be afraid to ask for help. It is really stupid to risk your reputation and the patient's well-being in order to prove bravado. People will trust you much more if they can rely on you to ask for help when necessary. In any case, seniors and nurses love showing off their skills.
• Wear gloves. The most unlikely people have Hep B.
• Remember that you can ask nurses for help in positioning and reassuring the patient.
• Use local anaesthetic for all but the smallest procedures.
• Keep a vial of atropine and a syringe to hand for procedures that involve puncturing serosal linings (pleura, peritoneum), as vaso-vagal events are reasonably common. Give one ampoule (0.6 mg) IV stat if the patient feels faint.
• Remember that you always have more time than you think, even during emergency procedures. If necessary hand your bleep to a nursing or medical colleague while 'scrubbed up'. Less haste more speed is a good maxim for invasive procedures.

Arterial blood gases

Bleeding tendency is a relative contraindication for taking ABGs. Ask a senior for advice if you are in doubt about whether or not to proceed. Always apply pressure for at least 5 minutes after taking ABGs from patients on warfarin or heparin.

Arteries in order of preference:

1 Radial—check collateral blood supply from the ulnar artery (especially if there is a history of wrist trauma) by asking the patient to make a tight fist and applying pressure over the radial artery. Ask the patient to relax the hand. If it remains white after 10 seconds, try the other arm.
2 Femoral—the problem here is that it is easy to hit the vein by mistake. Also, you really need to apply strong pressure to the puncture site for at least 5 minutes after taking blood.
3 Brachial—use this as a last resort. Use a 20–22 G needle. The femoral is easier as it is much larger and less likely to thrombose.

Have ready

1 Lidocaine.
2 One 2 ml syringe.
3 One 23–25 G needle.
4 Heparin (1000 U/ml).
5 Povidone or iodine swabs or alchohol swabs.
6 Sterile swabs/cotton wool balls.
7 Syringe cap (keep a personal stock, not all wards have these). Many hospitals supply special heparinized syringes, e.g. 'Pulsator' for taking ABGs.
8 Plastic bag or carton with a few ice cubes at the bottom.

The procedure (see Figs 13.1 & 13.2)

1 Ask your colleagues where the blood gas machine is and how to read it before taking blood (it is often in ITU or A&E).
2 Draw up 0.5 ml of heparin into a 2 ml syringe, withdrawing the plunger fully to coat the syringe walls. Expel the

heparin completely. You only need a few molecules to prevent the blood from clotting.
3 Wrist punctures are painful. It is a good idea to clean the skin and infiltrate superficially with a small bleb of local anaesthetic if there is no emergency.
4 Hold the syringe at a 60–90° angle to the skin and slowly advance the needle maintaining very slight negative pressure on the syringe. A flush of bright red blood indicates successful puncture. Keep very still and gently aspirate 1–2 ml.
5 Withdraw and apply pressure for at least 3 minutes (5 minutes if the patient is anticoagulated).
6 Expel all air from the syringe, tapping air bubbles towards the nozzle. Cap the syringe carefully and either take to the ABG machine immediately or place on ice and read as soon as possible (1 hour). Ice in a specimen bag is helpful to have ready so that you are not in such a panic to get to the ABG reading machine.

If you fail

• Re-direct the needle without coming out of the skin. Try aiming the needle at a more shallow angle. This allows a steadier approach. Withdraw and try again.
• If you hit bone, withdraw while gently aspirating.

Hints

• It is important to expel all the air from the sample. Once this is done ice only serves to slow cellular use of O_2 which is negligible over 60 minutes.
• Do not expect immediate ABG changes after adjusting someone's O_2

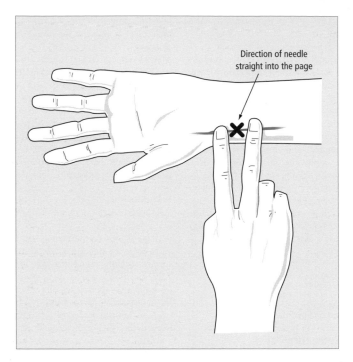

Direction of needle
straight into the page

Fig. 13.1 Radial arterial puncture.

supply. It takes up to 20 minutes for the ABGs to equilibrate to a change in inspired O_2 concentration. If a reading looks suspiciously high or low, repeat it.
• You can tell the difference between arterial and venous blood by its percentage saturation: 50% or less suggests venous blood, while 80% or above is certainly arterial.

Interpreting arterial blood gases

Normal ABG values are shown in Table 13.1.

Points to consider when interpreting arterial blood gases

For a full explanation of acid–base disorders consult any good medical textbook.

P_{O_2}

First ask yourself: does the patient have abnormally low O_2 for them? What is their baseline P_{O_2} value? Many patients with chronic respiratory disease live quite happily with a P_{O_2} of 7.5 kPa so don't get too flustered by an apparently terrible P_{O_2} value. Check the results of

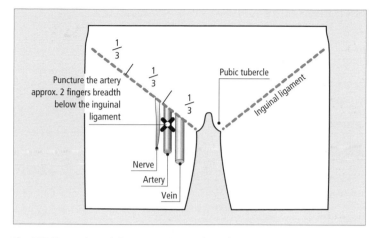

Fig. 13.2 Femoral arterial puncture: inguinal canal anatomy may be remembered using the mnemonic 'NAVY'—nerve, artery, vein, Y-fronts (!).

Table 13.1 Normal ABG values.

pH	7.35–7.45
P_{CO_2}	4.3–6.0 kPa
Base excess	± 2 mmol/l
P_{O_2}	10.5–14 kPa
Plasma HCO_3	22–26 mmol/l
O_2 saturation	95–100%

previous ABGs when the patient was well to see how much they have decompensated. (If you do not have any previous results to hand you may need to seek senior advice on how to proceed.)

Next check if the patient is retaining CO_2. This will determine the amount of O_2 therapy you can give (see p. 77).

Remember that the O_2 saturation curve for Hb is a steep sigmoid curve that starts to plateau around a P_{O_2} of 9.1 kPa (70 mmHg). This means a patient may

have a P_{O_2} of 8.5 kPa and still have better than 90% O_2 saturation. However, in the steep part of the curve (between P_{O_2} of 6 and 8 kPa), small changes in P_{O_2} dramatically affect O_2 saturation and are very clinically significant.

pH

Is it normal or is there an acidosis (pH <7.35) or an alkalosis (pH >7.45)? If either exists, decide if it is metabolic or respiratory and whether or not it is compensated (see Table 13.2).

A compensated acid–base disorder suggests more chronic disease, over days to weeks, while an uncompensated acidosis or alkalosis suggests a more acute disorder. In general, the body compensates for changes in pH by altering the respiratory rate (e.g. in metabolic acidosis, CO_2 is 'blown off') and regulating renal excretion of HCO_3. Except in

Table 13.2 Interpreting acid–base disorders

	pH	P_{CO_2}	HCO_3	K^+
ACIDOSIS				
Metabolic				
Early	↓	Normal	↓	Usually ↑
Compensated	Normal	↓	↓	Normal or ↓
Respiratory				
Early	↓	↑	Normal or ↑	↑
Compensated	Normal	↑	↑↑	
ALKALOSIS				
Metabolic				
Early	↑	Normal	↑	↓
Compensated	↑	Normal	↑↑	↑
Respiratory				
Early	↑	↓	Normal or ↓	↓
Compensated	Normal	↓	↓↓	Normal or ↑

Reproduced from Zilva J.F., Pannall P.R., Mayne P. (1989). *Clinical Chemistry in Diagnosis and Treatment.* Lloyd-Luke (Medical Books) Ltd, London.

acute illness, most acid–base disorders are compensated to some extent.

Serum electrolytes (Na, Cl and HCO₃)

If the patient is acidotic you will need to calculate the anion gap ([Na + K] – [Cl + HCO₃]) in order to refine the differential diagnosis. DKA, lactic acidosis, certain toxins and the acidosis associated with renal failure all cause increased production of unmeasured anions, resulting in an increased anion gap.

Hints

• When interpreting ABGs, do not forget to note if the patient is on O_2 and how much.
• A patient with a mixed picture or who is well compensated may have a normal pH. Check all the parameters of the ABG analysis, not just the pH and P_{O_2}.

• If the results of the ABG analysis are very poor, you may have sampled venous blood. This is likely if the percentage saturation is 50% or less. Percentage saturation of arterial blood is usually over 80%.
• Patients with decompensated organ failure (for example, cirrhosis, CCF, respiratory or renal insufficiency) may have developed acid–base and electrolyte disturbances over weeks. Do not be tempted to correct them in a day. Rather, try to get the patient a little better each day and review according to the time frame over which the patient's illness developed.

Respiratory disease and arterial blood gases interpretation

Type 1 respiratory failure (pink puffer):
• Pa_{O_2} less than 8.0 kPa (60 mmHg).

- Pa_{CO_2} less than 6.0 kPa (45 mmHg).
If stable, their ABGs will reveal a compensated respiratory alkalosis.

Type 2 respiratory failure (blue bloater):
- P_{O_2} less than 8.0 kPa (60 mmHg).
- P_{CO_2} greater than 6.0 kPa (45 mmHg).
If stable, their ABGs will reveal a compensated respiratory acidosis.

Bladder catheterization

Ask an experienced colleague to supervise your first attempt and ensure that you know the procedure before your first night call. Female nurses usually catheterize women; you usually have to catheterize men.

Men

Have ready

1 Catheterization pack—contains kidney bowl, gauze swabs, sterile towels, etc.
2 Sterile gloves.
3 Cleaning solution.
4 Sterile tube of lidocaine jelly.
5 10 ml syringe and 10 ml sterile water.
6 Several Foley catheters. For the first attempt, 14 G is the usual size. Use a silastic catheter (which is firmer) for problematic catheterizations or when long-term catheterization is anticipated.
7 Urine bag and stand.

The procedure

1 Get a clean trolley that has been swabbed with an alcohol swipe and place the catheter pack on it. Also get a catheter stand.
2 Wash your hands thoroughly.
3 Wheel the trolley to the patient's bedside, draw the curtains and fully expose the patient's penis. Make sure there are no bedclothes in the way that might dirty the working area. UTIs are easy to induce with catherization.
4 Tell the patient what you are about to do and why you are doing it.
5 Without touching the sterile contents themselves, open the catheter pack, sterile gloves, tube of lidocaine jelly, syringe, water and catheter onto the catheter tray (or a sterile surface). Pour the cleaning solution (some hospitals use sterile saline alone) into a receptacle.
6 Put on gloves.
7 Drape the sterile towels or paper sheets to leave only the patient's penis exposed.
8 Gently retract the foreskin and clean the urethral opening with cleaning solution, keeping one hand clean for inserting the catheter.
9 Gently squeeze the contents of the tube of lidocaine jelly into the urethra, massaging the underside of the penis to work the jelly towards the bladder.
10 Open the catheter wrapping at the tip end only and insert the catheter into the urethra, withdrawing the plastic covering in stages as you go. This is the trickiest part of the procedure. Make sure the end is in the kidney bowl to collect urine. You should get some urine back when you reach the bladder from all but the most dehydrated patients.
11 If you feel resistance, gently pull the shaft of the penis upwards. In some cases pulling the penis down between the legs is more useful. *Never* use force.
12 Once fully inserted, inflate the

catheter balloon with 5–10 ml of sterile water by placing the syringe directly over the proximal opening (no needle) and pushing hard. Stop immediately if the patient experiences pain, as the balloon may be in the urethra. Once inflated, gently pull the catheter until you feel resistance of the balloon so that you are sure that it is stable in the bladder.

13 Gently pull back the foreskin. If you cannot, gently try again. If the foreskin genuinely gets stuck and starts to swell, get senior help immediately. Paraphimosis is a medical emergency.

14 Connect the end of the catheter to the bag and mount on a catheter stand.

15 Briefly document the procedure in the notes and record any significant volume of urine (>10–20 ml) that was collected in the kidney dish in the patient's fluid chart, particularly if the patient is in renal failure.

16 Send a sample of urine for MC&S.

If you fail

• The catheter may be blocked with jelly. Aspirate the catheter with the syringe or gently massage the bladder above the pubic bone to encourage urine flow.

• The patient may have a large prostate or penile stricture. For strictures, a smaller size catheter should be used—proceed with care and be ready to abandon the procedure! For large prostates, *larger* catheters are useful, particularly stiff, silastic ones.

• If after several attempts with different size catheters you cannot access the bladder, never be shy of calling for help. Even the most senior urologists have trouble sometimes and can show you tricks for really difficult urethras.

• Supra-pubic catheterization is a useful last resort. Again, ensure supervision before attempting this alone as you risk perforating bowel.

Women

Have ready

Same equipment as for the men.

The procedure

1 Position the patient as for a vaginal examination. Ask her to lie flat on her back, knees bent, feet together and to allow her knees to fall down in full abduction.

2 Part the labia minora and clean the area with cleaning solution.

3 Locate the urethral opening just posterior to the clitoris and introduce a well lubricated catheter tip. Female catheterization is usually much less problematic than for males because they have no prostate and a really short urethra.

As you will probably only be asked to catheterize women that the experienced nurses cannot manage, get taught how to do this before you get called. Be aware of underlying causes for the problem such as tumours. If concerned, do a PV and do not be shy to call for help from a senior nurse.

Blood cultures

If you are going to the trouble of doing blood cultures it is better to do two sets from different sites, particularly if accurate diagnosis is very important. Three sets should be taken at 2–3 hourly intervals for suspected infective endocarditis.

Have ready

1 1 or 2 sets of culture bottles (some hospitals now use a single type of culture bottle for both aerobic and anaerobic cultures).

2 Two 20 ml syringes and needles.

3 Lots of alcohol swabs.

The procedure

1 Select a vein.

2 Clean the skin with alcohol, from the centre out. Allow to dry.

3 Without relocating the vein, cannulate and withdraw at least 10 ml of blood for each set of cultures.

4 Withdraw and inject at least 5 ml into each bottle.

5 Place in incubator as soon as possible.

Hints

• It is not necessary to change needles between taking blood and inserting it into the culture bottles. There is increased risk of needlestick injury and little increase in contamination.

• It is also unnecessary to clean flip-cap culture-bottle tops.

• The above technique is fine for easy veins. If not, use a dressing pack, iodine, swabs, etc., and scrub up after you have got the patient ready. Keep your gloves sterile, as this will allow you to palpate for veins

Blood letting

Have ready

1 Tourniquet.

2 Needles (green or blue).

3 Syringe(s) of adequate size for the bloods you need to take.

4 Alcohol swab(s).

5 Cotton wool ball or small plaster.

6 Blood tubes.

7 A sharps container.

Vacutainers are much quicker to use than needles and syringes but have no 'flash-back' to let you know when you have entered the vein. Therefore it is probably a good idea to use syringes and needles at first.

The procedure

1 Put on gloves.

2 Tell the patient what you are doing and why.

3 Choose the preferred arm (*not* a drip arm); tighten the tourniquet above the elbow and find a vein (see below). Visualize which way the needle will slide along the vein.

4 Swab the insertion area.

5 Put the needle on the syringe. Holding the patient's skin taut around the vein, gently but firmly advance the needle through the skin and subcutaneous fat into the vein. With practice you feel the vein give way when you are through. You should get a small 'flash-back' in the base of the syringe.

6 Holding the syringe and needle in the arm very still, steadily draw back the syringe until you have enough blood

7 Loose the tourniquet *before* withdrawing the needle.

8 Apply pressure to the puncture site with cotton wool or have the patient do so.

9 Taking care not to stick yourself, insert the needle into the blood tubes and allow the vacuum to withdraw the blood. (Some labs recommend that you remove

the needle from the syringe, uncap the tube, and gently squirt the blood directly into the tube. This prevents needlestick injuries. In practice, very few House Officers we know use this technique.) Never squirt blood into the tube through small needles as this risks haemolysis and false readings.

10 Tidy up, especially sharps.
11 Send blood to the lab.

Choosing a vein

Ask the patient for his or her preferred arm. Usually the left arm is best for right-handed patients. Obvious forearm or cubital fossa veins are good. In dialysis patients, never use their AV fistula arm.

If you can't find a vein

1 Hang the arm over the edge of the bed, 'milking' it or tapping the back of the hand.
2 Use a sphygmomanometer; it is better than a tourniquet. Pump it up to diastolic pressure, asking the patient to pump their hand. For problematic patients use a sphygmomanometer first off.
3 Immerse the arm or hand in a bowl of warm water for 2 minutes; pump the sphygmomanometer up with the arm in the water; dry the arm and quickly look for veins.
4 Pump up the sphygmomanometer to above systolic pressure, asking the patient to exercise the hand until it aches (1–2 minutes), then release the pressure to diastolic level. The lactic acid produced as a result of anaerobic metabolism is a potent vasodilator. This method is painful. Use as a last resort.

Hints

• Always gently invert filled tubes containing anticoagulant so that no clotting occurs (e.g. haematology tubes).
• For the same reason, don't over-fill heparinized tubes—they will clot.
• Paediatric tubes, which only require a few drops of blood, can be used for patients with very difficult veins.
• Find out from the labs how much blood is really necessary for standard tests at your hospital. Often you need very little.
• Try removing the rubber stopper of the bottle if you need to put more blood in the bottle and you have lost the vacuum. Gently squirt blood from the syringe directly into the bottle having removed the needle (to avoid haemolysis).

Cannulation (Venflon/line insertion) (see Fig. 13.3)

No matter how much of a klutz you think you are, you will soon be inserting cannulae with the best of them. Practice really is the only way to be good at this. Here we outline the basic procedure with a trouble-shooting guide; the best way to learn the procedure is to get someone to show you.

Have ready

1 Tourniquet or sphygmomanometer.
2 Appropriate size cannula (see Table 13.3).
3 Cannula dressing (wing-shaped).
3 5–10 ml syringe.
4 Saline flush.
5 Alcohol swab(s).

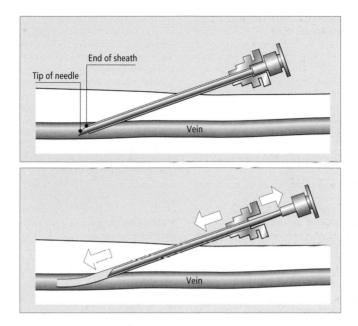

Fig. 13.3 Cannulating a vein.

Table 13.3 Cannulae sizes.

Colour	Size	Use
Blue	22 G	Small, fragile veins
Pink	20 G	IV drugs and fluid administration
Green	18 G	Blood transfusions, fluids
White	17 G	As above
Grey	16 G	Rapid fluid administration, GI bleeds
Brown	14 G	Very rarely used, major bleeds

6 Cotton wool ball/small plaster.
7 Bandage and tape.

The basic procedure

1 Put on gloves.
2 Tell the patient what you are doing and why.
3 Choose the preferred arm. Tighten the tourniquet above the elbow and find a vein (see below). Visualize which way the needle will slide along the vein.
4 Swab the insertion area and allow the alcohol to dry (or it will sting).
5 Firmly advance the needle through the skin and subcutaneous fat into the vein. With practice you feel the vein give way when you are through. You should get a small 'flashback' of blood in the base of the cannula.
6 Holding the cannula in the arm very still, withdraw the metal stylet and *simultaneously* advance the plastic cannulae into the vein.
7 Undo the tourniquet and secure the cannula with a dressing. It is a good idea to secure the cannula with a covering bandage to prevent it catching on bedclothes.
8 Tidy up, especially sharps.

Choosing a vein

1 Ask the patient for his or her preferred arm. Usually the left arm is best for right-handed patients. Remember that the dorsum of the hand is more convenient for you, but less so for the patient. Obvious forearm veins are good (in dialysis patients, never use their AV fistula arm).
2 Avoid sites where two vein joins are tethered. While these can be easier to cannulate, the drip is more likely to tissue as a result of poor flexibility.
3 Avoid foot veins except as a last resort. They thrombose more readily and are prone to infection.
4 Avoid crossing joints.
5 Shave hairy arms for ease of cannulation and to reduce pain when removing the drip.
6 Palpate the vein, visualizing which way the needle will run along it.
If you can't find a vein, see p. 147 (blood letting).

Hints

• Emla anaesthetic cream is extremely useful for squeamish patients. Keep a tube handy. Apply over selected veins and cover with an occlusive dressing. Simply wipe off in 30 minutes to 1 hour and site the drip as usual. Injection of local anaesthetic is less useful as it often obscures the vein.
• It is helpful to take blood at the same time as putting in the cannula. This must not be done with 'precious' veins. Once the cannula is secured, elevate the arm above the level of the left atrium. Remove the cap and place a syringe into the back of the cannula. Lower the arm (sometimes you need to reinflate the cuff gently) and *very gently* aspirate the required amount of blood (rapid aspiration causes the vein to collapse down in to the cannula). You may need to withdraw the cannula slightly, or lift the wings of the Venflon away from the skin a little way to initiate the flow of blood into the syringe.
• Pink, rather than green, cannulae are adequate for most routine purposes, such as saline infusions or IV drugs.

Saving a dying drip or cannula

When asked to re-site a cannula because it has tissued:

1 Ask whether or not it is still really necessary.

2 Many lines can be flushed gently with 5 ml of heparinized saline that clears any minor blockage. Small syringes (2 ml) are most effective at clearing minor blocks.

3 Always remove the cannula if the site is inflamed.

Times when a cannula MUST be in place, even at night

• The acutely ill or unstable patient.
• Hypovolaemia or poor oral intake.
• Serious danger of blood or fluid loss.
• Certain IV drug infusions—antibiotics, cardiac infusions, heparin, etc.

Central lines

Ensure that you are supervised for your first attempts; this procedure has the potential for some big time complications. The two most commonly used veins are the internal jugular and subclavian, usually on the right side. Other underused approaches include the femoral vein and the median basilic vein, both of which are technically easier but don't last as long. The same principles apply to all CVP lines. The jugular approach should be attempted first, as it has fewer complications, and it is easy to stop any bleeding, including arterial bleeding, should you miss. Having said that, the artery is palpable next to the vein, and therefore more easily avoided than with the subclavian approach. Unless you feel very confident with central lines, it is better to call for help than to attempt subclavian access yourself.

Indications for CVP lines

• Measurement of CVP.
• Infusing certain drugs and TPN.
• Inserting Swan-Ganz catheters or pacing wires.

Insertion of central lines

When to use the jugular approach

1 Clotting problems, typically when the INR is greater than 5 or the platelet count is less than $100 \times 10^9/l$.

2 Respiratory disease where a pneumothorax might be life threatening although they can still occur with this approach.

Have ready

1 Central line set.
2 Standard dressing pack.
3 Betadine.
4 Sterile gown and gloves.
5 One large sterile drape.
6 10 ml 1% lidocaine.
7 Two 10 ml syringes.
8 Heparinized saline (Hepsal) to flush lines.
9 25 G (orange) and 21 G (green) needles.
10 Suturing material (2-0 or 3-0 silk or prolene).
11 Scalpel blade.
12 Two adhesive dressings.
13 500 ml bag of saline and giving set.
14 CVP manometer.

The procedure (see Fig. 13.4)

1 Have the trolley ready (sterile contents laid out). Remove all pillows. Tilt the bed to lower the patient's head (to fill the neck veins). Tell the patient what you are about to do and why. Reassure them that while it is uncomfortable to lie still and backwards for about 20 minutes, that the procedure is not painful.

2 Wash your hands well and put on gloves.

3 Flush the giving set and CVP manometer with heparin saline.

4 Clean a wide area of skin from the inside out around the puncture site and cover with the drape.

5 Flush the central venous cannula and connecting tubing with saline.

6 Check that the guide wire passes through the large bore needle and determine which is the soft, 'vessel-friendly' end.

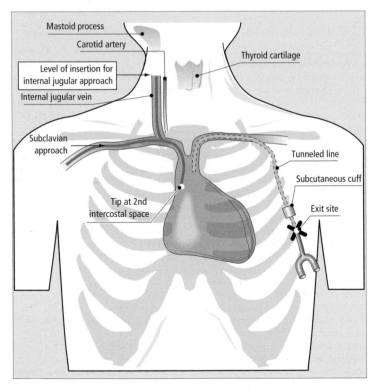

Fig. 13.4 Illustration of positions for insertion of central lines.

Cannulating the right internal jugular vein

1 Feel for the pulse of the carotid artery with the left hand. With the right hand, infiltrate local anaesthetic subcutaneously at the level of the thyroid cartilage and lateral to the carotid artery. Whenever you infiltrate with local anaesthetic, **always** aspirate while advancing to avoid injection into a blood vessel. Also remember that all vials look remarkably similar. Always take the time to check that you are drawing up the right stuff. (This may seem obvious, but it is easy to forget and regret!)

2 Whilst guarding the carotid artery with the left hand, insert a green needle attached to a 10 ml syringe, at an angle of 45° to the neck, heading towards the right anterior superior iliac spine. The right nipple in males is also a good landmark. Some line kits come with a cannula that is fitted over a needle (a bit like a big Venflon). This contraption can be attached to a syringe and directly advanced in the same way as the green needle.

3 Advance slowly, aspirating for blood. The vein is superficial. Do not go more than a few centimetres. If you fail to get blood, withdraw slowly, you may have gone through the vein. If this doesn't work, try again, slightly more medially. If by mistake you do hit the carotid artery, don't panic; apply strong pressure for 5 minutes

4 When you have entered the vein, withdraw the needle. Take the large bore needle with attached syringe and follow the line taken with the green needle. If using the cannula-over-needle supplied in the kit, then withdraw the needle alone once you have entered the vein, while advancing the cannula into the

vein, as you would a Venflon. Aspirate to ensure that the cannula is sited in the vein. Cap or occlude its open end to prevent air entry. The cannula is now ready to accept the guide wire (see below). Once the guide wire is threaded, the cannula may be withdrawn over the wire (remember never to let go of the wire while doing this).

Cannulating the subclavian vein

1 Visualize the sternoclavicular and acromioclavicular joints to find the intersection of the medial one-third and lateral two-thirds of the clavicle.

2 Beginning about 1 cm below the clavicle, infiltrate local anaesthetic right up to the clavicle, including the periosteum, using a blue needle.

3 Insert a green needle through the anaesthetized area and advance towards the clavicle, aiming for the suprasternal notch (see Fig. 13.4). Aspirate and infiltrate with local anaesthetic as you go. Once you reach the clavicle, work your way down it until the needle goes just under the inferior surface. You usually will not reach the vein with a green needle.

4 Repeat step 3 with the large bore needle, aspirating as you go. If you fail, aim slightly more upwards.

Inserting the guide wire

1 Before inserting the guide wire, ensure that you can aspirate blood freely through the needle.

2 Ask the patient to breathe out. As he or she is doing so, remove the syringe and place your thumb over the lumen to prevent air entry.

3 Insert the soft end of the guide wire.

It should pass with minimal resistance. *Never* force it. If it won't pass, check you can still aspirate blood and try again. If it still won't pass, change the angle of the needle slightly.

4 Pass about 50% of the length of the wire and remove the needle, holding the end of the wire firmly.

5 Nick the skin at the line's entry point with a scalpel blade. Thread the dilator and twist it down over the wire to the hilt. Remove the dilator, taking care not to pull out the wire, then thread the catheter. Remove the wire.

6 Check you can aspirate blood from each lumen of the catheter. Flush with heparinized saline (Hepsal) before clamping each lumen.

7 Secure with two sutures and place two occlusive clear dressings like a sandwich over the cannula.

8 Do a CXR to check the line's position and to exclude a pneumothorax.

Hints

• For the subclavian approach, placing a 1 l bag of saline between the patient's shoulder blades makes access easier.

• The breathless patient need only be flat or head down for cannulation of the vein and insertion of the guide wire. The rest can be done sitting up.

• Always take the pulse following the procedure. Frequent ectopics suggest the catheter is in the right ventricle and should be pulled back into the vein.

• If you hit the carotid or subclavian artery apply firm pressure for a full 5 minutes.

• Never attempt both subclavian veins without obtaining a CXR.

Problems with temporary and tunnelled central lines

You will often be called to sort out line problems. The commonest are:

Sepsis. If a patient with a central line develops a fever, take peripheral and central blood cultures. If the patient is clearly septic (temperature >38°C, tachycardia, pain/inflammation around entry site) discuss removing the line with your senior. Tunnelled lines can sometimes be treated with antibiotics if the patient is otherwise well, but this cannot be done for short term lines when the track is much shorter. After removal of any central line, always cut the tip off with a sterile pair of scissors and send it for culture.

Blocked lumen. This is prevented by daily flushing with heparinized saline (available on most wards in prepared vials). If the line is blocked, flush using a 1–2 ml syringe with heparinized saline, applying moderate pressure. Remember to put in a heparin–saline lock after flushing. Lines near the lumen sometimes wind around on themselves; simple unwinding can sometimes alleviate apparently severe blocks. If still no luck, a dilute solution of urokinase can be instilled by repeated aspiration and injection. Leave it for 30 minutes, then try flushing again.

Hints

• Taking blood from central lines should only be performed as a last resort. You need to discard the first 15 ml of blood and use a good aseptic technique. Do not take samples for aminoglycoside levels from a central line as these drugs are adsorbed by the cannula.

• A 1–2 ml syringe is more effective for unblocking cannulae than a 5 or 10 ml syringe.

Using central lines

Hickman and Groschong lines are tunnelled lines intended for long-term use such as for chemotherapy or TPN. Groschong lines have a special two-way valve system at the tip of each lumen that prevents blockage after flushing and facilitates taking of blood samples. However, the valve excludes the use of the line for CVP measurements. It is extremely useful to know how to handle these lines. Infection is the major problem and most patients are trained in looking after their own line. They are very critical of sloppy technique. Therefore, before handling a line, ask a nurse or medical colleague to give you a quick tutorial. The basic technique outlined below is a guide only. Different units use different IV connectors, bungs, etc. For setting up an IV, giving drugs or taking blood via a tunnelled line you will need to:

1 Open up:
   • Dressing pack.
   • Sterile gloves.
   • One 5 ml syringe and heparin–saline or saline.
   • One sterile luing (and plug for cannula).
   • Four alcohol swabs.
   • Cleaning solution, for example, betadine solution, and container.
2 Get an assistant (always handy).
3 Scrub up.
4 Keep one hand absolutely sterile.
5 Handle the line with dry sterile gauze.

6 Remove the bung from the end of the line using a swab and discard.
7 Always open and shut the gate or clamp between procedures.
8 Attach drip or take bloods as appropriate.

Measuring the CVP (see Fig. 13.5)

The CVP is measured with reference to a fixed point, either the mid-axillary line or the manubriosternal angle. The pressures at the manubriosternal angle will be about 5–7 cm lower than those at the mid-axillary line. It does not matter which you use, as long as you remain consistent.

1 Lie the patient flat. Adjust the scale so that the 10 cm mark is opposite the chosen reference point (marked with an indelible pen). If you use the true '0 cm' level you cannot measure negative values.
2 A three-way tap controls the flow of fluid between the IV bag, the CVP reading scale and the patient. Adjust the tap to run fluid from the bag up to the 30 cm mark on the manometer. Set the tap to connect the patient to the manometer. The manometer fluid level should swing with respiration and settle. The CVP is measured in cm of water.

Hints

1 Learn to measure the CVP yourself and take the time to ensure that nursing staff are familiar with doing CVP measurements. It is easy to get it wrong.
2 Normal values for CVP:
   Using the 10 cm mark aligned with the manubriosternal angle: 7–14 cm.
   Using the 10 cm mark aligned with the mid-axillary line: 11–18 cm.

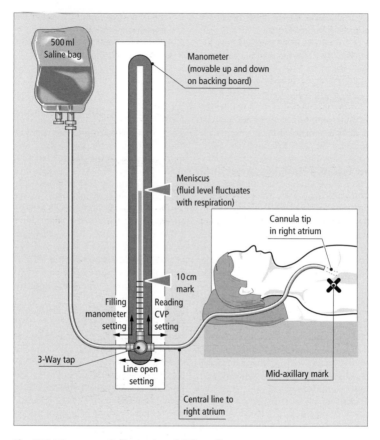

Fig. 13.5 Diagrammatic illustration of CVP reading.

(Subtract 10 cm if using the true 0 cm mark.)

3 The CVP reading should be regarded with suspicion if right atrial pressure is likely to be abnormal:

• Raised intrathoracic pressure (tension pneumothorax).

• Altered intravascular volume (fluid overload or hypovolaemia).

• Abnormal venous tone (NB catecholamine release can maintain CVP readings despite significant blood loss). Other drugs can cause dramatic loss of tone and drops in CVP.

• Abnormal right ventricular function: CCF, pericardial tamponade/constriction, acute RVF. The CVP may be markedly raised following right-sided AMI or large PE. The CVP in these situations is an unreliable guide to fluid status. If called to see a patient with a rising or falling CVP think of the above approach to guide you.

Chest drains

You are unlikely to be expected to insert chest drains, but you will be expected to manage and remove them. The decision to remove a drain should be taken by your seniors. The following paragraphs give general guidelines for maintaining and removing drains (see Fig. 13.6).

Indications

Pneumothorax.
Haemothorax or empyema.
Large pleural effusion.

Managing a chest drain

Pneumothorax

1 Check for an air leak by asking the patient to cough. A bubbling drain

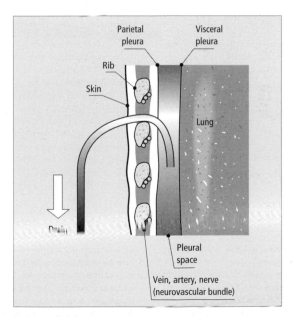

Fig. 13.6 Cross section through chest cage to illustrate chest drain.

implies an air leak from an unsealed hole, fistula or a leak in the tubing. You may need to apply suction to the drain if you suspect a hole or fistula.

2 After the lung has re-expanded and the drain is no longer bubbling, clamp and re-X-ray. If there is no pneumothorax and the fluid is cleared, the drain can be removed.

Effusion/haemothorax

1 Large effusions can drain over several days, up to a maximum of 1 litre/hour and not more than 4 litres/day (otherwise there is a risk of 'reflex' pulmonary oedema). Remove the drain when the CXR reveals no further fluid.

2 For recurrent effusions you may consider chemical pleurodesis; discuss with your team.

3 Empyema drains require special consideration. Get a specialist opinion.

How to remove a drain

Have ready

1 Gloves.
2 Clamping forceps.
3 Pair of scissors.
4 One occlusive dressing.

The procedure

1 Clamp the tube with the forceps.

2 The entry point of the tube should have been secured with a purse-string suture that must be untied (not cut) and the ends firmly pulled to seal the hole as the tube slides out. Take your time the first few times you do this. It is easy to lose the stitching.

3 Withdraw the tube with positive intra-thoracic pressure by asking the patient to blow hard against a closed nose and mouth ('Make your ears pop'). You should hear the hiss of the expulsion of the last bit of air as the end comes out. Quickly pull the purse string to seal the hole. Apply an occlusive dressing.

4 Do a CXR to assess the success of the drain and as a comparison for future X-rays.

Hint

Have a 4 × 4 cm gauze swab to hand to place over the hole in the event of a failed purse-string closure. Later, replace this with a large clear occlusive dressing over the hole.

DC cardioversion

As a House Officer rotating through cardiology, you may be asked to do the elective cardioversion list for patients in stable atrial fibrillation. This may seem daunting, yet it is a straightforward procedure, providing the patient has been adequately prepared (see p. 122).

1 Once the patient has been anaesthetized, ask the anaesthetist whether he/ she is happy for you to continue.

2 ENSURE THAT THE DEFIBRILLATOR IS SET TO 'SYNCHRONIZED'. Check that the defibrillator is sensing QRS complexes rather than T or P waves. You may need to adjust the gain to achieve this.

3 Apply gel pads over the right sternal edge and over the cardiac apex, avoiding the nipple (since the skin is much more sensitive, and does not take well to having current passed through it).

4 Set defibrillator to 100 J.

5 Warn all present that you are about to charge the paddles, and make sure everyone is standing clear (you will note that the anaesthetist will withdraw to a safe distance, taking the patient's oxygen mask with him or her).

6 Press the paddles firmly onto the pads on the patient, charge them up, and deploy the shock. From the time you press the button to administer the shock, there may be some delay before the shock is deployed. This is because the defibrillator is waiting for the next QRS complex. During this delay, do not be tempted to think the paddles have not worked, and take them away prematurely.

7 Replace the paddles and check ECG or rhythm monitor. (Once the paddles have been replaced, the anaesthetist will continue ventilation.)

8 If the procedure has not worked, repeat at 200 J. If this too does not work, repeat at 360 J. Check the gel pads between each shock to make sure that they have not dried out, as this will lead to skin burns.

9 If, at 360 J, the procedure has not caused reversion to sinus rhythm, consider repositioning the paddles, with one at the left sternal border, and one to the left of the spine at the same level, and administering another 360 J shock.

10 At the end of the procedure, do a formal 12 lead ECG, and ensure patient is in the recovery position, and is still ventilating well, with good oxygen saturation.

Hints

Do not be too hasty in judging whether a treatment cycle has been successful or unsuccessful on the basis of the rhythm monitor. It may take a few seconds for the rhythm to settle into sinus after a shock, and, likewise, the initial appearance of sinus rhythm may give way to atrial fibrillation within a minute or so.

Electrocardiogram

Many indications, especially history of IHD; DM; hypertension; SOB; chest pain; swollen leg; pre-op. ECGs don't take much time and are harmless; if in doubt, just do one.

The procedure

1 Have the patient lie with their chest exposed. Explain to them what you are doing and reassure them that there is no way that they will get an electric shock.

2 Attach limb leads to the inner aspect of the forearm just below the wrist and the outer aspects of the leg above the ankle. The wires are usually labelled but if not the colour code is most often as follows:

    Red = right arm
    Yellow = left arm
    Green = left leg
    Black = right leg

3 Ensure good contact with electrode jelly (you can also use K Y jelly)

4 For chest leads see Fig. 13.7.

Hints

• Doing ECGs is mostly a hassle when you don't know where to find a portable ECG machine. To save sleep, make sure you know where one is before you go to bed, as well as where you can find re-

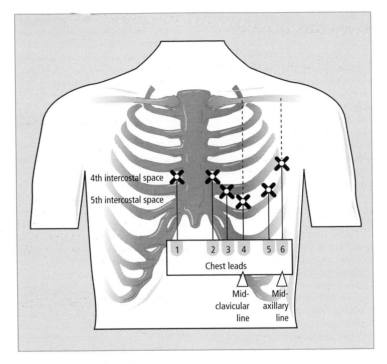

Fig. 13.7 ECG chest lead placement.

placement paper, electrode jelly or disposable electrode pads for the lucky few hospitals that have them.

Preventing spurious results:
• The patient should be completely relaxed. Explain that the procedure is completely painless and harmless.
• Make sure the chest lead electrodes do not overlap.
• Lightly shave very hairy areas for proper contact.
• If the patient has a hand tremor (e.g.

Parkinson's) attach the leads higher up the arm.
• The black (right leg) lead is an earth lead and can be attached to any part of the body. It has no bearing on the result.
• For leg amputees, the green (left leg) lead can be placed on either leg. However, the arm leads must not be crossed. For an arm amputee, ensure that the arm electrodes are equidistant from the heart (they may be placed on the shoulders).

Reading ECGs (see pp. 52–55)

Exercise stress test

Exercise (ECG) stress tests take approximately 20 minutes to perform. Your job is to encourage the patient to attain their peak heart rate if possible (= 220 – patient age), and to watch their ECG closely. Your aim is to detect and measure the severity of coronary artery disease, and to uncover arrhythmias.

Relative contraindications (discuss with senior)

Aortic stenosis.
Hypertrophic obstructive cardiomyopathy.
LBBB on ECG.
Systolic BP >200 mmHg; diastolic BP >100 mmHg.
Unstable angina.
Uncontrolled arrhythmias.
Note: Beta-blockers should be stopped 2 days before the test.

The procedure

1 Make sure that there is resuscitation equipment immediately available. Approximately 1 per 4000 patients arrests during stress tests. Also have GTN ready.
2 Known peak heart rate = 220 – patient age.
3 Follow the instructions of the ECG technician, who has followed the protocol many times.
4 *Stop the test* if the patient complains of:
  • Increasingly severe chest pain or other symptoms (such as faintness or dyspnoea). Consider administering GTN.
  • A fall in systolic BP of more than 20 mmHg.
  • A fall in heart rate.
  • VT or VF.
  • Progressive ST elevation.
  • ST depression greater than or equal to 2 mm.
  • Three or more consecutive ventricular ectopics.
  • Peak heart rate is attained.
5 You must remain present at all times and monitor BP and pulse at regular intervals (ask the technician for local protocol). This includes the recovery period when the test may become positive, or (horrors) the patient may go into VT. (Be ready to resuscitate.)

Glucose tolerance test

Indications

Suspected diabetes mellitus.

Have ready

1 The patient should have fasted overnight.
2 75 g oral glucose dissolved in a glass of water.
3 Apparatus for taking blood with grey (glucose) tube.

The procedure

1 Take a fasting sample for blood glucose in a grey tube.
2 Give the patient the oral glucose with the water to drink over less than 5 minutes.

3 Take a second blood glucose sample after 2 hours.

Interpreting the results

1 Normal result: 2 hour glucose level is less than 7.8 mmol.
2 Impaired glucose tolerance: fasting plasma level less than 7.8 mmol and the 2 hour level between 7.8 and 11.1 mmol.
3 Diabetes confirmed: fasting plasma level greater than 7.8 mmol and the 2 hour level greater than 11.1 mmol.

Injections

Subcutaneous

Have ready

1 23–25 G needle.
2 Alcohol swab.

The procedure

1 Choose a fatty site and use the smallest possible needle.
2 Clean site with an alcohol swab and allow to dry.
3 Gently pinch a wad of skin and fat between your thumb and index finger.
4 Place the needle on the skin for 3 seconds at an angle of about 60° before pushing through the skin. This reduces the sensation of pain. Release the skin.
5 Aspirate to ensure you do not inject into a blood vessel.
6 Slowly depress the plunger. Rapid injection will cause pain.
If you aspirate blood, remove and replace the needle and explain to the patient the need to repeat the injection.

Intramuscular

Have ready

As for SC.

The procedure

1 The deltoid muscle is usually good for small injections. If the patient is thin or wasted use the gluteal muscles—choose the upper and outer quadrant below the iliac crest to avoid the sciatic nerve by drawing an imaginary line between the anterior superior iliac spine and the greater trochanter of the femur, and injecting posteriorly to and above this line (see Fig. 13.8).
2 Pull the skin taut and inject at 90° to the skin (pulling the skin ensures that the injection doesn't leak after you pull the needle out).
3 Aspirate to ensure you do not inject into a blood vessel. Inject slowly.

Intercostal block

Indications

Very effective for severe, localized, pleuritic chest pain (e.g. localized pleuritis, metastases, fractured ribs). Intercostal blocks usually abolish pain and surprisingly the relief lasts longer than the action of the anaesthetic.

Have ready

1 Dressing pack and sterile gloves.
2 Betadine.
3 One 10 ml syringe.
4 One 23 G needle.
5 One 21 G needle.

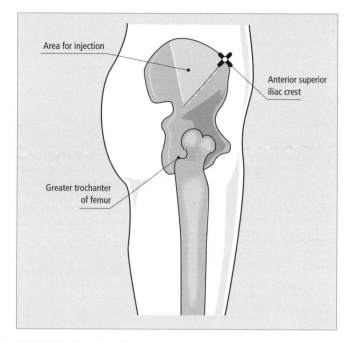

Fig. 13.8 Site for intramuscular injections.

6 5–10 ml 2% lidocaine or 0.5% bupiva-caine (preferred, because it is longer acting).

The procedure

1 Identify the interspace(s) where the pain is arising and the spaces above and below. Prepare the skin in the mid-axillary line. Anaesthetize the skin using a 23 G needle just below the inferior margin of the rib with lidocaine. You need to deliver the drug close to the nerve.

2 Change needle to 21 G (green). Going through the same puncture site, advance at an upward angle again towards the inferior margin of the rib. The nerve lies inferiorly in the groove. If you hit bone, withdraw slightly and try again, slightly more inferiorly. Aspirate to ensure the needle is not in a vessel and slowly inject 1–2 ml of bupivacaine.

3 Repeat the procedure for the inter-spaces above and below.

Joint aspiration/injection

This is useful procedure to learn from an expert, especially if you are an aspiring

GP. Superb aseptic technique is vital as is a sound knowledge of the anatomy. Each joint requires a slightly different approach but the basic technique is the same.

Aspiration

Indications

Diagnostic:
• Recent onset arthritis.
• To rule out infection (acute and chronic).
• Joint effusion.
Therapeutic:
• Steroid injections.
• Drainage of septic arthritis.

Have ready

1 Three syringes (5, 10 and 50 ml).
2 Two needles (25 G and 21 G).
3 Lidocaine 2%.
4 Sterile gloves.
5 Sterile dressing pack.
6 Betadine solution.
7 Three specimen containers and a fluoride tube (grey top) for infections.

The procedure

1 Written consent is advisable.
2 Find the site of maximal effusion and mark this point with indelible ink.
3 Scrub up and clean the area with betadine. Allow it to dry and wipe over the site of aspiration with an alcohol swab. Allow it to dry completely. Even small amounts of betadine will ruin your culture results.
4 Anaesthetize the area being careful to avoid injecting local anaesthetic into the joint—lidocaine is also bactericidal so will mess up cultures.
5 Insert the aspiration needle and advance it slowly whilst maintaining slight negative pressure. When you hit the effusion, tap it completely.
6 Never inject steroids if joint infection is a possibility. To inject steroids after tapping an effusion, disconnect the syringe leaving the needle in place. Attach the syringe containing the steroid. Aspirate to ensure you are not in a vessel, then inject. There should be minimal resistance. Stop if you feel you are in the tissues and try again.
7 Remove the needle and apply pressure for a minute. Dress the wound.

Hints

• Phone microbiology to request urgent microscopy on the joint fluid. Some labs insist on special transport media when certain infections are suspected—get advice from the microbiologist.
• The sub-talar joint (below the ankle joint) is notoriously difficult to aspirate—get expert help.

Injecting joints

Many rheumatology departments teach a simple no-touch technique. The risk of infection following this method is no worse than that outlined above.

Have ready

1 Two 5 ml syringes—one for lidocaine (to anaesthetize the skin) if deemed necessary, and one for the steroid, ± lidocaine.
2 Two alcohol swabs.

3 A small plaster.

4 Triamcinolone (5–20 mg) or methyl-prednisolone (10–40 mg) for steroid injections. The dose will depend on the size of the joint.

The procedure

1 Inform the patient of the small risk of infection (see above).

2 Draw up the lidocaine (if required) and the steroid for injection. The latter is now available with lidocaine added. This limits the potentially painful response to the injection and lasts about 2–3 hours. Note that the lidocaine for skin anaesthesia is still advisable for squeamish patients.

3 Locate the site for injection; clean with an alcohol swab and allow to dry. Without touching the site again push through the skin and anaesthetize the skin down to the joint. Remember to aspirate to ensure you are not in a vessel. Remove and allow a minute for the local anaesthetic to work.

4 Repeat (3) except this time inject the joint with steroid. There should be minimal resistance to the injection.

5 Remove the needle and apply pressure for a minute. Dress the wound.

Hints

• Tell the patient that mild pain and redness can occur after steroid injections and may persist up to 48 hours. They are due to a reaction to the crystalline suspension used in long-acting steroids, but be wary of iatrogenic infection.

• Never inject steroids if joint infection is a possibility.

Local anaesthesia (for any procedure)

Have ready

1 21 G and 23 G needle.

2 5–10 ml syringe.

3 Alcohol swabs.

4 1–2% lidocaine ampoules.

The procedure

1 Start with a 23–25 G needle. Infiltrate the skin and SC tissues raising a small bleb. If deeper anaesthesia is required, switch to a larger needle (21 G), wait 1 minute, then pass through the same puncture site.

2 Aspirate for blood before injecting anything. If you hit blood, withdraw a little and try again.

3 Wait at least 2 minutes for effect.

Hints

• Lidocaine lasts approximately 2 hours. Marcain and bupivacaine are longer acting (8 hours) and useful for intercostal blocks.

• Use lidocaine with adrenaline for very vascular sites where you need to incise skin, as adrenaline causes vasoconstriction. *Never* use adrenaline for a nerve block of an extremity, e.g. a finger, nose block.

• To work out the dose of lidocaine in mg/ml, multiply the percentage concentration by 10. Maximum dose of lidocaine within 24 hours:

　Without adrenaline: 3 mg/kg

　With adrenaline: 7 mg/kg

Lumbar puncture

Lumbar punctures are actually pretty easy once you get the hang of them. The thing to do is to reassure the patient that it is an uncomfortable but relatively painless procedure, and that it might take up to 30 minutes—so you don't feel rushed. Of all procedures, this one requires a slow, methodical approach for success.

Indications

Diagnostic:
• Meningitis, SAH, rarities.
Therapeutic:
• Intra-thecal drugs (never to be given by House Officers—a job for SHOs and above).

Contraindications (get help)

1 Local sepsis.
2 Raised ICP (vomiting, bradycardia, drowsiness, papilloedema).
3 Suspicion of a cord or posterior fossa mass.
4 Coagulopathy or platelet count <40.
If patient is drowsy, unconscious or has evidence of raised ICP, request an urgent CT scan before doing an LP.

Have ready

1 LP pack or if none available:
2 Two sterile drapes.
3 One gallipot.
4 One pack gauze swabs.
5 One pack of cotton wool balls.
6 Two LP needles (an 18 G (yellow) or a 20 G (black); open one).
7 One sterile, disposable manometer.
8 Three sterile, 20 ml specimen containers.
9 Antiseptic (povidone/betadine solution or equivalent).
10 5–10 ml lidocaine 2%.
11 10 ml syringe.
12 23 G and 21 G needles.
13 Sterile gloves.

The procedure (see Fig. 13.9)

1 Obtain oral consent. Explain to the patient what you are doing, that the procedure may take some time but is not very painful—just uncomfortable.
2 Ask the patient to lie as indicated in Fig. 13.9a—with knees tucked up under the chin as much as possible (to draw the spinal cord out of the way of the needle). Ensure the vertebral column is parallel to the bed (the hips are exactly perpendicular to the edge of the bed).
3 Get an LP pack ready on a trolley with plenty of room to manoeuvre. Make room for sharps and dirty items.
4 Scrub up as for a sterile technique.
5 Prepare skin with betadine and cover with a sterile drape.
6 Unscrew the tops of the three sterile sample containers.
7 Locate the puncture site L3–L4 or L4–L5 by drawing two imaginary lines, one joining the top of the iliac crests and the other running down the spine. These intersect at L3–L4. The spinal cord ends at L1–L2, so the L2–L3 interspace is safe if you cannot use the lower interspaces for some reason, but ensure the patient is properly curled up.
8 Anaesthetize using a 23 G needle for superficial skin and SC infiltration. Switch to a 21 G needle for deeper infiltration into the interspinous ligament.

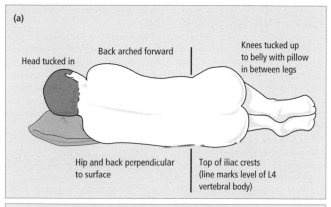

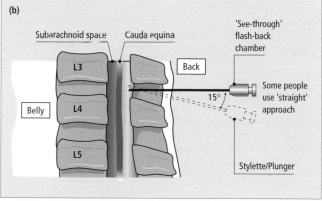

Fig. 13.9 (a) Patient position for lumbar puncture. (b) Approaches for lumbar puncture.

Inject slowly waiting at least 2 minutes for effect.

9 Assemble the LP equipment, check that the stylette moves freely within the needle, and check how to use the manometer taps.

10 Insert the needle in the midline between the two spinous processes. Advance towards the patient's umbilicus (slightly towards the head). Resistance increases as the needle passes through the interspinous ligament. A small 'give' is felt as the needle punctures the ligamentum flavum. Withdraw the stylette to check for a flash back of CSF. If there is no CSF, advance the needle a few millimetres and check again.

11 Attach the manometer, allow the

patient to relax and measure the pressure (recorded in cm H_2O; normal range 6–15 cm). The level will fluctuate with respiration.

12 Disconnect the manometer. From the open end of the needle collect:

- 2–5 drops for biochemistry.
- 5–10 drops for bacteriology.
- Up to 5–10 drops for cytology.

13 Withdraw the needle slowly, taking care not to spill too many drops of CSF (causing a severe headache afterwards). Dress the wound.

14 The patient should lie flat for 4 hours. They may have a moderate headache afterwards. If they experience a severe headache they should inform the nurses or doctors.

If you fail

- Correct positioning is the key to success. If you fail, re-check the patient's position. Try another interspace if necessary.
- If the patient is anatomically 'difficult' (e.g. very large or has an abnormal spinal column), ask a more experienced senior or enlist the help of a radiologist who can do the LP under X-ray screening.
- You feel you are in the right place but no CSF—lightly rotate the needle through 90°; the bevel may be lying against a nerve root.

Hints

- Sedate the patient if required: 2.5–5 mg diazepam orally 30 minutes before the procedure. The patient needs to remain horizontal for at least 4 hours post-LP to reduce the incidence of severe headache. Warn the patient that

headaches can occur up to 3 days after an LP.

- *Never* apply suction to a CSF needle.
- Subarachnoid haemorrhage is easily distinguishable from a bloody tap by uniform blood staining of the three consecutive samples and xanthochromia in the supernatant. The samples from a bloody tap gradually clear. Send samples for a cell count.

Mantoux test

Indication

A Mantoux tests for a delayed-type hypersensitivity reaction to a partially purified protein derivative from *Mycobacterium tuberculosis*. For routine pre-BCG skin testing the 10 unit dose of tuberculin PPD is used.

Have ready

1 Order PPD from pharmacy.
2 1 ml diabetic syringe (26 G 1 cm needle).
3 Alcohol swab.

The procedure

1 Dilute PPD to a concentration of 100 TU/ml.
2 Draw up 0.1 ml (10 TU) into a diabetic syringe.
3 Clean a small area on the left forearm (convention).
4 Indicate the area to be injected with a marker pen.
5 Keeping the needle almost horizontal to the skin, carefully insert the needle intra-dermally and inject 0.1 ml so that a small bleb is raised.

6 A negative reaction at 48 hours indicates a negative response.

7 Read at 72 hours. Measure the diameter of induration, not the erythema:

- >10 mm = positive; suggestive of previous or current infection, not necessarily disease.
- >20 mm = strongly positive, highly suggestive of active disease.

Nasogastric tubes

Nurses are usually experienced at inserting NG tubes; you are usually called only if they fail. Therefore it is a good idea to do a few before such a call. They are usually straightforward.

Have ready

1 An apron and non-sterile gloves.
2 Fresh NG tube—size 10 (small) to 16 (large).
3 Kidney bowl and catheter drainage bag.
4 KY jelly.
5 Glass of water.

The procedure

1 Sit the patient upright with chin on chest.
2 Tell the patient what you are doing and ask for their help in swallowing the tube.
3 Lubricate the tube with jelly and insert into a nostril. Gently advance the tube towards the occiput (not upwards). Ask the patient to swallow when they feel the tube at the back of their throat and advance the tube as they swallow. They may find swallowing the water simultaneously to be helpful.

4 To assess position: aspirate some contents using a small syringe and test with blue litmus paper to check the contents are gastric (blue litmus paper turns red on contact with acidic gastric juices); or, with a syringe, blow air down the tube whilst listening with a stethoscope over the stomach.

5 Attach the drainage bag.

If you fail

- Try the other nostril.
- Try oral insertion—ask the patient to swallow the tube.
- Sometimes NG tubes have two lumens. If you don't block off one lumen when syringing air through the other to check the position of the NG tube, it will appear (falsely) as if the tube is not in the stomach.
- Get help from a senior.
- Consider endoscopic placement under mild sedation.

Hints

- NG tubes are uncomfortable and predispose to sinusitis. Remove as soon as possible.
- Use fine-bore tubes for enteral feeding.

Peritoneal tap (paracentesis)

Like pleural aspiration, paracentesis is remarkably straightforward and even quite fun. The procedure is identical to pleural aspiration except for the position of the patient and puncture site.

The procedure

1 Ask the patient to empty their bladder. Explain what you are doing and why. Stress that the procedure is painless except for initial anaesthesia.
2 Lie the patient as flat as possible.
3 Percuss out the ascites.
4 Scrub up, prepare the skin and drape.

Give local anaesthetic in the sites indicated in Fig. 13.10.
5 Follow the same procedure as for pleural aspiration (see below).
6 For therapeutic taps use a suprapubic or peritoneal dialysis catheter. These are usually supplied with drainage bags.
7 Send samples for biochemistry (protein, glucose, LDH), bacteriology

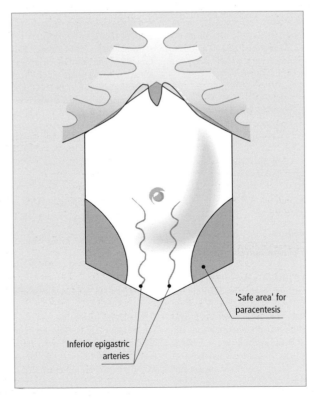

Inferior epigastric arteries

'Safe area' for paracentesis

Fig. 13.10 Site for tapping ascites.

(MC&S, ZN stain and TB culture) and cytology.

Hints

• Do not remove more than 500 ml in the first 10 minutes and no more than 1200 ml in 24 hours. Removing more fluid risks hypotension but may be appropriate for some patients; check with your senior.

• Avoid going too close to old surgical scars as bowel may be attached to the abdominal wall.

• You may need to reposition the catheter or 'jiggle' the patient to maintain the flow.

• Bizarre cells on cytology often represent reactive mesothelial cells, not malignancy. Always get a formal report before embarking on a hunt for a tumour.

• Complications are rare but include perforated bowel, peritonitis, intra-abdominal haemorrhage and perforated bladder.

• Paracentesis is essential to rule out peritonitis in patients with cirrhosis and long standing ascites who become decompensated.

Pleural aspiration

Pleural aspiration is straightforward, although the idea of plunging tubing into someone's chest sounds daunting. Ask a senior nurse or medical colleague to supervise your first one.

Indications

Diagnostic:
• Infection.
• Malignancy.

Therapeutic:
• Large effusions for relief of SOB.

Have ready

1 Dressing pack (some hospitals have a prepared pleural aspiration pack).
2 Sterile gloves.
3 One 10 ml syringe.
4 One green needle.
5 One blue needle.
6 10 ml 2% lidocaine.
7 Three specimen jars (sterile).
For therapeutic taps add:
8 One large bore IV cannula (brown or grey Venflon).
9 One three-way tap.
10 IV giving set and an empty, sterile bowl or saline bag.

The procedure

1 Confirm the size and extent of the effusion on the most recent CXR. Scrub up. Tell the patient what you are doing and how long it will take.

2 Sit the patient upright in bed or sit them on a stool leaning slightly forward over the side of the bed, resting their elbows on a pillow.

3 Select the insertion site by tapping out the effusion. The best sites are usually two to three spaces below the lowest point (angle) of the scapula or at the same level in the posterior axillary line. Avoid the mid clavicular line on the left (the heart!).

4 Scrub up and drape as for a sterile procedure. Ensure you have a sterile, flat surface on which to put things.

5 Anaesthetize the skin first with a 23 G (blue) needle for superficial infiltration and then again with an 18 G (yellow) needle for deeper infiltration. The track

of the needle should hug the upper border of the rib to avoid the neurovascular bundle (Fig. 13.11). Always withdraw before injecting local anaesthetic to make sure you are not in a blood vessel. In the average person, you should aspirate pleural fluid at the full depth of a green needle.

6 Attach a 20 ml syringe to the end of a green needle and insert the needle through the area already anaesthetized. Aspirate as you push forward. The flash back of fluid indicates that you have reached the effusion.

7 Gently aspirate 20 ml of fluid for analysis. Send for:

- Bacteriology: MC&S, ZN stains and TB culture.
- Chemistry: protein, glucose, LDH and amylase.
- Cytology—the more fluid the better (up to 10 ml) as the sample is spun down to concentrate the cells.

8 For therapeutic taps attach a large (white/brown/grey) cannula to a 50 ml syringe and after the flash back of fluid, advance the Venflon slightly and withdraw the needle, leaving the flexible cannula in place. As you do this, ask the patient to breathe out, placing your thumb over the cannula lumen to prevent air being sucked in. Again, ask the patient to breathe out as you attach the three-way tap. Secure the cannula with tape if you are aspirating a large effusion. Attach the 50 ml syringe to one tap, the empty saline bag to the other.

9 Aspirate 50 ml at a time, switching the tap settings to empty the syringe contents into the bowl or saline bag. Do not remove more than 1000 ml at one

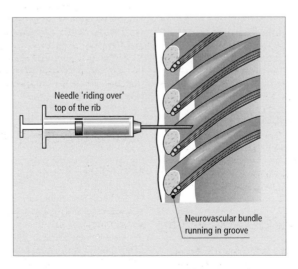

Needle 'riding over' top of the rib

Neurovascular bundle running in groove

Fig. 13.11 Pleural aspiration (diagram shows an oblique section).

sitting; more than this can lead to reflex pulmonary oedema.

10 Withdraw the cannula asking the patient to breath out as you do so. Apply an occlusive dressing.

11 CXR is usually only necessary if you have removed a large volume of fluid (>500 ml) or you are concerned about a pneumothorax.

12 Document the procedure, including the macroscopic appearance of the fluid (straw-coloured, blood stained, containing pus), the volume aspirated, and if you have done (and checked) a CXR.

If you fail

A dry tap indicates a possible loculated effusion or empyema. Try redirecting the needle. If no luck, ask for help from a colleague or radiologist.

Hints

• Ask the patient to cough as you reach the end; this aids in expelling fluid. They usually cough reflexly as the visceral pleura touches the end of the cannula.

• Have a vial of atropine to hand for vaso-vagals (1 ampoule (0.6 mg) IV stat).

• A 'pre-med' of pethidine (50 mg) IM and prochlorperazine (12.5 mg) IM is very useful for anxious patients.

• Do not take diagnostic samples from the giving set bag (if you use one) as it probably contains a filter that will exclude cellular material.

Pulsus paradoxus

During inspiration, intra-thoracic pressure falls, which reduces the systolic ejection volume and therefore the systolic pressure. Normally, the difference in the systolic pressure during inspiration and expiration is less than 10 mmHg. This pressure difference is exaggerated by a large drop in intra-thoracic pressure that occurs during inhalation in serious conditions, including severe asthma and cardiac tamponade. Pulsus paradoxus is defined by a difference in systolic BP between inspiration and expiration of more than 10 mmHg.

Have ready

A stethoscope and a sphygmomanometer.

The procedure

1 Inflate the cuff above systolic pressure, then slowly deflate until the first, intermittent sounds are heard (during expiration). Note the pressure.

2 Continue to deflate the cuff slowly until the sounds are continuous (i.e. heard during inspiration and expiration). The drop in mmHg between when the first sound is heard (intermittent) and when it becomes continuous represents the degree of paradox.

Respiratory function tests

Spirometry

Have ready

A spirometer, vitalograph paper and a disposable mouthpiece.

The procedure

1 Explain the procedure to the

patient and that you need their co-operation.

2 Plug the machine in. Place the vitalograph paper in position on the spirometer. Make sure the spirometer's needle is set to zero. Place the disposable mouthpiece in the end of the spirometer's hosepipe.

3 Ask the patient to take a couple of deep breaths. When ready, ask them to breathe in as deeply as possible and then to breathe all the way out as quickly as possible into the mouthpiece. They should breathe out until the needle reaches the end of the graph paper.

4 Depending on how automated the machine is, you may need to push the record button while the patient is exhaling.

Table 13.4 Expected values for FEV_1 (litres).

(a) Males

Age (years)	Height (m)				
	1.50	**1.60**	**1.70**	**1.80**	**1.90**
15–20	2.80	3.30	3.55	3.90	4.30
20–25	3.25	3.60	3.95	4.35	4.70
25–35	3.10	3.45	3.80	4.20	4.55
35–45	2.80	3.15	3.50	3.90	4.25
45–55	2.50	2.85	3.20	3.60	3.90
55–65	2.15	2.50	2.90	3.25	3.60
65–75	1.85	2.20	2.60	2.95	3.30
75–80	1.55	1.90	2.25	2.65	3.00
85+	1.40	1.75	2.10	2.50	2.85

(b) Females

Age (years)	Height (m)				
	1.40	**1.50**	**1.60**	**1.70**	**1.80**
15–25	2.45	2.80	3.15	3.45	3.75
25–35	2.35	2.65	2.95	3.30	3.65
35–45	2.05	2.35	2.65	3.05	3.35
45–55	1.75	2.05	2.35	2.75	3.05
55–65	1.45	1.75	2.10	2.45	2.75
65–75	1.15	1.45	1.85	2.15	2.45
75–80	0.85	1.20	1.55	1.85	2.15
85+	0.75	1.05	1.35	1.70	2.05

5 Repeat a few times, particularly if the first attempt(s) are feeble.

6 Record the best FEV_1 and FVC in the notes, with expected values for the patient (see Tables 13.4 & 13.5):

The patient has a restrictive picture if FVC is reduced and FEV_1/FVC >75%.

The patient has an obstructive picture if FEV_1/FVC <75%.

Peak expiratory flow rate

Measures the maximum expiratory flow rate in the first 2 ms of expiration, and is useful for assessing the respiratory status

Table 13.5 Expected normal values for FVC (litres).

(a) Males

Age (years)	Height (m)				
	1.50	1.60	1.70	1.80	1.90
15–20	3.45	4.00	4.50	5.05	5.55
20–25	3.65	4.15	4.70	5.20	5.75
25–35	3.55	4.05	4.60	5.10	5.60
35–45	3.30	3.85	4.35	4.90	5.40
45–55	3.10	3.60	4.15	4.65	5.20
55–65	2.85	3.40	3.95	4.45	4.95
65–75	2.65	3.15	3.70	4.20	4.75
75–80	2.45	2.95	3.45	4.00	4.50
85+	2.35	2.85	3.35	3.90	4.40

(b) Females

Age (years)	Height (m)				
	1.50	1.60	1.70	1.80	1.90
15–25	2.90	3.40	3.85	4.35	4.75
25–35	2.75	3.25	3.70	4.15	4.55
35–45	2.45	2.95	3.45	3.90	4.35
45–55	2.20	2.65	3.15	3.60	4.05
55–65	1.90	2.35	2.85	3.30	3.75
65–75	1.60	2.10	2.55	3.00	3.45
75–80	1.30	1.80	2.25	2.70	3.20
85+	1.20	1.65	2.10	2.60	3.05

of patients with asthma, COAD and other respiratory conditions, especially before surgery.

Have ready

A peak flow meter and disposable mouthpiece.

The procedure

1 Put the disposable mouthpiece into the peak flow meter.
2 Ask the patient to breathe in as deeply as possible.
3 With their lips tightly sealed around the mouthpiece, ask them to blow out

Table 13.6 Predicted values for PEFR (litre/minute).

(a) Males

Age (years)	Height (m)				
	1.50	**1.60**	**1.70**	**1.80**	**1.90**
15–20	440	475	510	545	580
20–25	535	570	610	645	680
25–35	525	560	595	630	665
35–45	500	535	570	605	635
45–55	480	510	545	575	610
55–65	455	490	520	550	580
65–75	435	465	495	525	550
75–80	410	440	465	495	525
85+	410	430	455	480	510

(b) Females

Age (years)	Height (m)				
	1.50	**1.60**	**1.70**	**1.80**	**1.90**
15–25	360	395	435	470	510
25–35	350	385	420	460	495
35–45	325	365	400	440	475
45–55	305	345	380	420	455
55–65	285	320	360	395	435
65–75	265	300	340	375	415
75–80	245	280	315	355	390
85+	235	270	305	345	380

Table 13.7 When to remove sutures.

Area sutured	Removal time (days)
Face and neck	3–5
Scalp	5–7
Abdomen and chest	5–10
If impaired wound healing (steroids, cachexia, severe infection, etc.)	14 or more

forcefully and quickly. Note the value attained.

4 Have them repeat it at least three times.

5 Record the best value in the notes, with the expected value (Table 13.6).

Sutures

You may be expected to do simple suturing. The method is best learnt in A&E or in theatre. Ask someone to teach you how to tie a basic, non-slip knot as soon as you can. Table 13.7 discusses times for suture removal.

Materials

1 Non-absorbable:
   • Nylon (ethilon).
   • Ethibond.
   • Prolene.*
   • Silk.*
2 Absorbable:
   • Plain cat gut (5–10 days).
   • Chromic gut (10–20 days).
   • Vicryl (60–90 days).*
   • Dexon (60–90 days).*

3 Sizes:
   • Very coarse—2, 1, 0, 1/0, 2/0, etc. Very fine—6/0, 5/0, etc.
   • 3/0 and 4/0 are suitable for skin on arms and legs.
   • 5/0 and 6/0 for face and back of the hand.
   • 2/0 is most often used for securing lines and 1/0 for chest drains.
4 Needles:
   Either use a cutting needle (with a bevelled edge) for suturing skin or a non-cutting needle (with a rounded end) for adipose and other soft tissues.

Hints

• Nylon is less comfortable for patients. Use softer, non-absorbable material (silk or prolene) for securing lines and chest drains.
• Some synthetic sutures are made as mono- or polyfilament. Monofilament sutures are more slippery, but are better if there is a high risk of infection. Polyfilament sutures facilitate tracking of fluid down the suture, leading to infection.

*Most commonly used for house officer purposes.

Chapter 14: **Radiology**

Radiologists can help you a great deal with patient management if you give them enough information.

Most of the following guidelines come from the Royal College of Radiologists. Your hospital may also have its own.

Requesting investigations

The task of requesting investigations is often delegated to House Officers. You will receive no end of grilling from overstretched radiology staff as to why this scan or that unusual view is needed. It saves a lot of time and hassle if you can supply cogent answers, so don't be shy to ask your seniors why *precisely* the investigation is needed. Besides which, you might learn a lot from asking.

1 Always book procedures as early as possible. Most radiological departments are overbooked. This is particularly true for contrast studies, CTs and MRIs.

2 Include lots of information on the X-ray form, such as:
  • Patient ID.
  • Whether pregnant or not. Any reactions to contrast media.
  • Whether patient is *C. difficile* or MRSA positive.
  • A specific question to be answered.
  • Clinical features (not just suspected diagnosis).
  • Any factors which may complicate the procedure (for example, diabetes, epilepsy).

  • 'Please' and 'Thank you' go a long way.

3 Ask the radiographers about how to prepare patients for investigations, such as barium enemas. Often the radiographer will liaise directly with the ward nurse, in which case you don't have to do anything except prescribe preparations, such as enemas (see p. 182). It can be good, however, to find out about the different preparations so that you can tell patients in advance what they are letting themselves in for. Better still, try them yourself—you will never order a barium meal lightly again!

Minimizing radiation

• 27% of the radiation we are exposed to comes from radiological sources.

• In terms of radiation, different procedures are ranked as indicated in Table 14.1.

Common concerns about X-rays

Patients are usually concerned about being X-rayed. It is much kinder to address their likely concerns outright. Therefore, wherever possible, tell the patient:

1 What is about to happen to them.

2 Why they are having this done.

3 How long it might take.

Table 14.1 Radiation doses of radiological investigations.

Investigation	Radiation dose (mSv)	Number of CXRs
Abdomen	1.5	75
Barium–oesophagus study	2	100
Barium–small bowel study	6	300
Barium–stomach study	5	250
Biliary tract	1.3	65
Cervical spine	0.1	5
Chest film	0.02	1
CT chest/abdomen	8	400
CT head	2	100
Dorsal spine	1.0	50
Extremities (e.g. knee)	0.01	0.5
Hip (one)	0.3	15
IVU	4.6	230
Large bowel study	9	450
Lumbar spine	2.4	120
Nuclear study bone	3.8	190
Nuclear study kidney	0.7	35
Nuclear study liver	0.7	35
Nuclear study lung	1.2	60
Nuclear study myocardium	18	900
Nuclear study thyroid	1	50
Pelvic plain film	1	50

RCR Working Party (1998). *Making the Best Use of a Department of Clinical Radiology: Guidelines for Doctors*. 4th edn. The Royal College of Radiologists, London.

4 Whether or not they will be sedated or have a general anaesthetic.

5 The amount and type of pain and discomfort to expect.

6 What to do if they have pain or other symptoms after the procedure.

7 When they can eat/drink/drive/talk/have sex.

8 Whether they will have any scars or permanent after effects.

9 Who is doing the procedure.

Pregnancy

• Referring clinicians (i.e. you) are responsible for informing the radiologist if a patient is pregnant. Notify the radiologist clearly on the X-ray form. It is negligent not to do this. Where possible tell the radiologist yourself.
• If you need to X-ray a pregnant patient, ask the radiologist for advice; they may suggest an alternative. Irradiation between the knees and diaphragm should be avoided.

Plain films

Chest X-rays before surgery

'Routine' CXRs are warranted pre-operatively if the patient has:
• Chronic heart or lung disease and no CXR within 12 months.
• Acute respiratory symptoms.
• Known/suspected malignant disease.
• Possible TB.
Age, smoking and mild hypertension are *not* reasons for routine chest X-rays.

Checking the CXR: the bare bones

1 Patient's name and the date of the film.
2 Trace the diaphragm and the lateral outline of the rib cage (? pleural effusions, air under the diaphram, raised hemi-diaphragm, pneumothorax).
3 Check the size and shape of the heart (? enlarged heart, atrial shadows, calcified valve rings).
4 Check the position of trachea and heart (? displaced or is the film rotated).

5 Look at the mediastinum (? air, widened, lymphadenopathy).
6 Examine the hilar shadows (? enlarged pulmonary arteries and veins).
7 Examine the lungs (? opacities—consolidation, fluid or nodules). For interstitial oedema remember to look for straight lines (normal interstitial shadows are 'never' straight).
8 Check the bony structures (ribs, clavicles, spine) and the soft tissues (fractures, densities or lucencies, air in the tissues).

Skull X-rays

You rarely need to X-ray someone's skull following a head injury. A CT is the investigation of choice. The Royal College's guidelines are shown in Table 14.2.

To differentiate CSF from normal nasal or aural discharge in a patient with head injury, test it with a urine dipstick. CSF contains glucose.

Abdominal films

Radiation dose: 75 CXRs.
Preparation:
• None.
Tell the radiologist:
• Presenting symptoms (not just 'acute abdomen').
• Past surgery.
• Pregnancy.
• Ask for an erect film if you need to check fluid levels.
Tell the patient:
• Quick, minimal irradiation.
A decubitus film is an alternative to an erect CXR to see perforation if the patient is too ill to sit up.

Table 14.2 Royal College guidelines regarding skull X-rays.

SKULL X-RAY NOT INDICATED	MANAGEMENT
All of the following: • Full orientation • Neurologically normal • No scalp laceration or haematoma • Amnesia <10 minutes	• Request neurological observation 6-hourly from the nurses (if already an inpatient) *or* have relatives take home a head injury form

SKULL X-RAY OR CT INDICATED	MANAGEMENT
Full orientation plus any one or more of following: • Serious scalp laceration • Scalp haematoma (90% are associated with fracture) • Clinical signs of closed fracture • Known loss of consciousness • Amnesia <10 minutes • Evidence of foreign body • Evidence of penetrating injury	• CT is the investigation of choice. Unless you are expert at reading skull X-rays show a skull X-ray to a senior before going to bed

SKULL X-RAY OR CT	MANAGEMENT
One or more of the following: • Disorientated or worse • Difficult to assess; drunk	• Admit for observation • Consult with neurosurgeons if fracture evident *or* no improvement in 12 hours

RCR Working Party (1998). *Making the Best use of a Department of Clinical Radiology: Guidelines for Doctors*. 4th edn. The Royal College of Radiologists, London.

Checking an abdominal plain film

1 Patient's name and date of the film; whether taken erect, supine (usual) or lateral decubitus.

2 Gas pattern; intestinal diameter: small bowel >2.5 cm, or colon >6 cm indicates obstruction.

3 Look for ascites and soft tissue masses ? Oedema in the intestinal wall. Fluid distribution.

4 Identify the liver and spleen.

5 Check the borders of the kidneys, bladder and psoas muscles if possible.

6 Calculi (gall stones, renal and pancreatic calculi, aortic calcification).

7 Sub-diaphragmatic gas (or clear outline of organ) indicates perforation or recent surgery. (Note: sub-diaphragmatic gas is best seen on an erect CXR. The absence of free gas under the diaphragm does not rule out perforation.)

Contrast studies

Intravenous urography

Radiation dose: 230 CXRs.
Preparation:
• Picolax (1 sachet) 12–24 hours before the procedure (not essential).
• Preferably NBM 6 hours before.
• Keep well hydrated before and after, to minimize contrast nephrotoxicity; give IV fluids if necessary.

Tell the radiologist:
- If patient has renal damage, diabetes or myeloma.
- Contrast allergy or pregnancy.

Tell the patient:
- Warn about preparation.

Barium swallow

Radiation dose: 100 CXRs.
Preparation:
- NBM 6 hours before.

Tell the radiologist:
- Oesophageal disease or surgery.
- Contrast allergy or pregnancy.

Tell the patient:
- Quick, painless but tastes horrible!

Barium meal

Radiation dose: 250 CXRs.
Preparation:
- NBM 6 hours before.

Tell the radiologist:
- Upper GI disease or surgery.
- Contrast allergy or pregnancy.

Tell the patient:
- Painless but tastes awful.

Small bowel enema

Radiation dose: 300 CXRs.
Preparation:
- 24 hours low residue diet.
- Laxative (for example, 1 sachet of Picolax) 24 and 12 hours prior to procedure *unless* contraindicated (for example, IBD, PR bleeding); get radiologist's advice.

Tell the radiologist:
- Past surgery.
- Contrast allergy or pregnancy.

Tell the patient:
- Warn them about diet and laxative.

- Takes at least half an hour; may take 2 hours.
- Uncomfortable; requires upper GI intubation.

Barium enema

Radiation dose: 450 CXRs.
Contraindication:
- Severe colonic inflammation (for example, IBD, severe diverticulitis) and toxic megacolon.

Preparation:
- Do not perform immediately prior to CT abdomen/chest (barium hides detail on CT for at least 72 hours). Do the CT first or consider using gastrograffin.
- Book for >72 hours after rectal biopsy and rigid sigmoidoscopy to avoid perforation.
- Strong laxative 24 and 12 hours before procedure *unless* acute IBD; ask radiologist for advice.

Tell the radiologist:
- Previous surgery.
- Contrast allergy or pregnancy.
- Result of sigmoidoscopy/rectal biopsy/rectal exam.

Tell the patient:
- Warn them of diet and laxative.
- Procedure takes 20–30 minutes.
- Pictures will be taken every 10–15 minutes while the patient is turned around on a platform. The procedure is *very* undignified, uncomfortable and often upsetting.

Ultrasound

No radiation or contraindications.
Preparation:
- Abdominal US: NBM 6 hours before.
- Pelvic US: Requires full bladder.

• The patient should start drinking a few hours before the procedure.
Tell the patient:
• No radiation dose or known hazards; painless, relatively quick.

Computerized tomography

Preparation:
• Nil unless contrast is needed — ask the radiologist.
Tell the radiologist:
• Any metalwork *in situ* (difficult to interpret).
Tell the patient:
• Will be confined in a noisy tube.
• Painless; will be told what to do by the doctor and nurse.

General

• CTs give large radiation doses (400 CXRs equivalents for abdominal and chest CTs and 100 for skull CTs). Does the patient really need one?
• Usually hospital CTs are overbooked, so book your patient in as early as possible.
• Do CTs *before* requesting barium studies. Barium hides detail on CT and takes at least 3 days to clear. Gastrograffin can be used instead of barium if this is a problem.
• Patients may require sedation before CT. 10mg of temazepam 10 minutes before the procedure is usually adequate.

CT head — indications

Stroke: diagnosis in doubt; atypical clinical course; to differentiate haemorrhage from infarct if planning anticoagulation.

Must be done within 2 weeks for accurate differentiation.

Sub-arachnoid haemorrhage: to exclude a raised ICP before doing an LP; for diagnosis; to diagnose the cause of deterioration (re-bleed, hydrocephalus, vascular spasm).

Head injury: skull fracture and serious scalp injury; impaired consciousness, focal neurology; epilepsy; persistent confusion; deteriorating conscious level; depressed skull fracture; open skull fracture of vault or base.

Arteriography

Preparation:
• Nil to eat for 6 hours before; nothing to drink 3 hours before.
• G&S; FBC (specifically platelets); INR; find both femoral pulses.
• Keep well hydrated before and after to minimize contrast nephrotoxicity; give IV fluids if necessary.
• If patient has renal damage, diabetes or myeloma, discuss with radiologist.
Tell the radiologist:
• Contrast allergy or pregnancy.
Tell the patient:
• The radiologist will numb the skin in the groin and then inject some dye into the artery. They may get a bruise.
Risks:
1 3% chance of femoral puncture site damage (major haemorrhage requiring surgery or transfusion).
2 0.5% risk of occlusion of the artery or pseudoaneurysm.
3 2% risk of unintended occlusion of selected vessel.

4 0.5% risk of distal embolism.
5 0.1% risk of arteriovenous fistulae.
If there is angioplasty and/or stenting,
risks of the above all increase slightly.

Magnetic resonance imaging

• MRI does not emit ionizing radiation
but scans are expensive. Does your
patient really need one?
• Book your patient in as early as
possible and discuss the procedure with
radiologist.
• Inform the radiologist and get his or
her advice if the patient has a pacemaker,
metal heart valves or other metallic implants. Many modern implants are now
'MRI safe,' although you will need to
check the make with the radiologist.
• T1 weighted images give good anatomical detail. Fat is white, flowing blood
is black. T2 images are good at showing
abnormal tissue but have poor anatomical detail. Fat and fluid are bright.
Preparation:
• Sedation may be necessary (usually
given by the radiologist).
Tell the radiologist:
• If the patient is pregnant.

• Discuss with the radiologist if the
patient has any metal implants. **Do not
allow the patient to be scanned
unless you are certain that any implants are MRI-safe.**
Tell the patient:
• No irradiation is used. The procedure
is painless.
• The patient will be in a noisy, confined space for approximately 25 minutes, although it may seem longer.

Radioisotope scanning

Use to detect:
1 Bony metastases and sites of inflammation—technetium (Tm) scanning.
  • Radioisotope scanning delivers
  variable radiation doses. Ensure that
  the patient is not pregnant.
  • Most scanning does not require
  preparation, but as usual, book early.
2 Pulmonary embolism—ventilation
perfusion (VQ) scans.
  • There is no preparation for a VQ
  scan. These may only be available on
  certain days of the week, so make sure
  you book one well in advance.

Chapter 15: **Surgery**

Looking after surgical patients is not intrinsically difficult, but it does involve a lot of running around. You will accompany surgeons on many rapid ward rounds weekly. Have a piece of paper ready for the tasks that will be fired at you from all directions. Overall, the essential thing is timing—if nothing else, make sure you have patients and results ready for theatre.

Fluid chart.
Blood bottles and forms: (FBC, C&E, G&S or cross-match, ±INR ± glucose).
IV cannulae.
• Find out how to order sticky labels and order them whenever they look like they are running short on a patient. Writing patient details on endless forms and bottles is no fun.

Routine clerking

House Officers need to make sure that patients are fit for surgery. While clerking routine surgical patients can be mundane, it is useful to bear in mind that you may be the only one able to detect medical problems before the patient goes to theatre.
• *Before you see the patient*, quickly flick through the notes (summaries are particularly useful) to give yourself an idea of what has happened previously. This will reassure the patient and helps you to fill in their past medical history.
• Clerking patients before nurses have finished their admission routine is silly to create havoc. Ask the nurse to let you know when he or she has finished.
• Take everything you need to finish clerking to the bedside:
    Sticky labels.
    History sheets (see right).
    Consent form.
    Drug chart.

History sheet
1 Operation (for example, 'For TURP'), last meal, LMP
2 Past surgical history
3 Past medical history (HASH CREDIT*)
4 Medications and CASES†
5 In women of child bearing age, ask for the date of their last menstrual period and whether they may be pregnant.
6 *Allergies* (very important—especially past drug reactions to anaesthesia)
7 Home care (lives with, home help, family, allowances, mobility)

continued on p. 186

* HASH CREDIT: **H**ypertension, **A**sthma/COAD, **S**ickle cell, **H**IV/Hepatitis, **C**VA, **R**F, **E**pilepsy, **D**iabetes, **I**schaemic Heart Disease, **T**B. Alternatively, SHIRC DEATH, HEH DRASTIC.
† CASES: **C**ontraception, **A**nticoagulants, **S**teroids, **E**toh/alcohol, **S**moking.

continued on p. 186

8 Functional enquiry: CVS, RS, GIT, GU, CNS, MSK
9 Examination
10 Impression
11 Differential diagnoses
12 Plan

• Make your own protocol clerking sheet, custom-designed for your specialty (see Fig. 15.1, p. 187). If useful, include the boxed pre-op anaesthetist checklist (p. 192). To photocopy the protocol onto real history sheets, write or type it out on a blank sheet of paper lined up with a history sheet, and then feed real history sheets into the photocopying machine.

• If you have literally 3 minutes to clerk a patient, at least make sure that: (a) the patient has the problem that they are supposed to have; (b) they are fit for surgery. You may be the only person that checks them for cardiovascular and respiratory problems.

• G&S or cross-match patients ahead of time. It is wise to routinely G&S virtually all patients on admission if you have not already cross-matched them. If necessary you can then phone the blood bank to cross-match them quickly (in 30 minutes). Unless you ask the lab to hold onto it for longer, G&S blood is usually thrown out after 3 days and may need to be repeated (see Table 15.1).

• Check local transfusion requirements for specific operations.

• ITU can be a frightening place. Try to organize for patients undergoing major operations to meet ITU staff or visit the ITU before theatre in preparation for their post-op stay. Nurses will often organize this for you.

• Do a sickle cell test on black patients if their haematological status is unknown.

• Patients must be NBM for solids for at least 6 hours before going to theatre, and 3 hours for sips of liquid. This is a fairly strict rule. In a real emergency anaesthetists do 'crash induction'. Discuss this if necessary with the anaesthetist.

Perioperative prescribing

• Prescribe as much as possible during the clerking, as it saves time later: regular drugs; pre-medication; prophylactic antibiotics; prophylactic heparin; analgesia; routine post-op antibiotics (consider PR administration to save IVs); extra steroids if the patient takes them already (to overcome post-op stress).

• Check the firm's use of prophylactic antibiotics and anticoagulants.

• 20 mg temazepam orally with a small sip of water can be used as a pre-med if necessary. This can usually be given within an hour of theatre, although it should be given 3 hours before. Check with the anaesthetist if in doubt.

• A fentanyl infusion can be effective pain relief (less side effects than morphine but more expensive; problems appear within first 10–15 minutes).

• Patients should have stopped taking non-steroidals and anticoagulants *at least* a week (preferably a month) before surgery. If they have not, ask your senior

Name: .... DOB: .... Occupation: ....

Admitted for: ....

HPC: .... ☐ Weight loss ☐ Past PU
.... ☐ Change in bowel habit ☐ Alcohol intake
.... ☐ Blood in stool ☐ Smoking
.... ☐ Abdominal pain

Last meal: .... Last menstrual period: ....

PMH .... ☐ H/T ☐ RF
.... ☐ Asthma/COAD ☐ Epil.
.... ☐ Sickle ☐ DM
.... ☐ HIV/HEP ☐ IHD
.... ☐ CVA ☐ TB

Drugs: .... **Allergies:** ....
....

F/SHx: .... ☐ Lives with ☐ Family diseases
.... ☐ Home help ☐ Mobility

F/E ....

R/CVs	☐ Chest pain	☐ Cough w/y/g/sputum	☐ Palps
	☐ SOB	☐ PND	☐ Pillows
	☐ Dysuria	☐ Frequency	☐ Incontinence
GU	☐ Urgency	☐ Stream	☐ Haematuria
	☐ Froth in urine		
CNS	☐ Fits/faints/funny turns	☐ Change in vision/speech	☐ Weakness
D/MSK	☐ Joint pain	☐ Rash	

Other ....

Examination P = ... Reg/irreg .... BP = .../......
T = ... RR = ...

General	**R/CVS**	**Abdomen**	**Legs**
☐ Jaundice	☐ JVP	☐ Bowel sounds	☐ SOA
☐ Pallor	☐ Apex	☐ Tender	☐ Ulcers
☐ Cyanosis	☐ Bruit	☐ Mass	☐ Skin changes
☐ Lymphadenopathy	☐ Expansion	☐ Bruit	
☐ Plethora/oedema	☐ Breath sounds	☐ Shifting dullness	
☐ Clubbing	☐ PN	**CNS**	
☐ Rash	☐ SOA	☐ Reflexes ☐ Plantars ☐ Strength	
☐ Arcus	☐ HS	☐ Co-ordination ☐ Sensation	

Impression ....

Differential diagnosis ....

Plan ....

Fig. 15.1 Surgical protocol clerking sheet.

Table 15.1 Preparations for different operations.

Operation	G&S/cross-match	Special needs
Abdominoperineal repair/ AP resection	4	Prepare for stoma
Amputation (minor)	G&S	Pain ± grief
Amputation (major)	2+	Fentanyl and clonidine infusion works well; buscopan helps muscular contracture pain
Aneurysm repair (elective)	6	Post-op ITU
Aneurysm repair (emergency)	10	Post-op ITU
Aortobifemoral repair	6	
Appendicectomy	G&S	Metronidazole PR post-op saves a drip
Arthroscopy	Nil	
Carotid endarterectomy	2	
Cholecystectomy	G&S	
Colectomy	2	Prepare for stoma
Dynamic hip screw	2	Be alert to post-op infection
ERCP	G&S	Pre-op abdominal US Post-op amylase
Femoropopliteal repair	2	
Gastrectomy	2	Bad pain post-op; try continuous morphine infusion
Hemi-arthoplasty	2	
Hernia	Nil	
Ileal reservoir	2	
Laparotomy	2	Consent for colostomy/ileostomy
Liver biopsy	G&S	Pre-op INR (see p. 186)
Liver/pancreatic surgery	6	Post-op amylase
Mastectomy	G&S	Prepare for grief over loss of breasts and body image and get a prosthesis nurse to talk to the patient Drains in for several days (remove when they have stopped discharging)
Oesophagectomy	4	

continued

Table 15.1 (continued)

Operation	G&S/cross-match	Special needs
Prostatectomy (TURP)	2–4	Watch for post-op haemorrhage (look for bad haematuria). May need to cross-match more blood post-op
Pyloric stenosis	G&S	
Splenectomy	2	Pre-op pneumococcal ± HiB, ± meningococcal vaccines
Thyroidectomy	2–4	Pre op vocal cord assessment from ENT clinic post-op Ca check
Total hip replacement	4	Watch for DVT/PE and infection; usually routine anticoagulation required
TURT	G&S	Pre-op MSU
Varicose veins	G&S	

or anaesthetist for your firm's policy on how to proceed. The effects of anti-coagulants fall within days of stopping them and usually you can cover patients with FFP. Patients with artificial heart valves or other conditions requiring continuous anticoagulation should be switched over to heparin—consult your seniors.

• The *BNF* recommends that people stop taking the oral contraceptive pill at least 4 weeks before major surgery. If the patient has not done this, consider IV or SC heparin before surgery but discuss with the anaesthetist or surgeon first. The pill does not need to be stopped for minor surgery such as laparoscopic ster-ilization. Progestagen-only pills do not need to be stopped. In people who have stopped or have not been using contra-ception, exclude pregnancy. Consider a formal pregnancy test.

Consent

Criteria for valid consent*
1 No coercion
2 Patient informed
3 Patient competent

However rushed you are, patients must understand major and common hazards and discomforts of the procedure they are about to undergo (ideally you may only obtain consent for a procedure you have personally performed. How-ever, the situation 'on the ground' is very different and seniors often expect you to

* Hope R A. *et al.* (1994). *Oxford Practice Skills Project: sample teaching materials*. Oxford Medical School, Oxford.

'take consent'. Refuse except to give the patient information in advance of the operator getting informed consent (to make their job easier).

• If you will perform the procedure yourself (like a bone marrow biopsy), never get consent if you do not know all the risks or logistics of the procedure. If in doubt ask you senior.

• While taking consent, you can spend a few minutes improving the patient's understanding of their overall course of management (not just the procedure). This is a good opportunity to develop a relationship with the patient.

• A signature alone does not stand in a court of law as adequate proof of consent. The patient must understand the procedure.

• Make sure you get parental consent for minors while the parents are on the ward, or you will have to call them in from home. ('Minors' are people under 16 years of age.) Occasionally it may be lawful to treat a child under 16 without parental consent, but you must be sure that he or she fully understands the treatment, that his or her health would be likely to suffer without treatment, that you have attempted to persuade the child to involve their parents, and that you are sure it is in the child's best interest to proceed without informing the parents. You must get senior advice in these situations. Rarely, parents refuse consent to treatment that their child needs. Unless it is an acute situation, an application will be necessary through the hospital's solicitors or Social Services.

• Diagrams can save many words. If you are in a specialty where you need consent for a particular procedure many times, a well-constructed diagram can save you a lot of time in the long run. Photocopy it and leave it with the patient.

• Remember that while *you* may understand anatomical diagrams, the patient may not. Sometimes a conceptual diagram is more useful, if not as accurate. See Appendix B for diagrams which you can use to explain standard procedures to your patients.

• Check with nurses to see if your department has information sheets already made up which you can give to patients.

• Always consent patients undergoing laparoscopic surgery for open surgery. (5–10% of patients undergoing laparoscopic cholecystectomy end up having open surgery.)

• Always consider consenting patients undergoing bowel resection or laparoscopy for colostomy/ileostomy in case they need one. (Write '± colostomy/ileostomy' on the consent form.) Warn them that this may happen and arrange with the nurses for a stoma nurse to see them.

In all cases of surgery it is important to inform patients of:

• Fatigue. It is important to tell patients to expect to feel quite low and very tired for several weeks post-op (1–3 months for major surgery).

• Anaesthetic risk. Although the anaesthetist will consent for the anaesthetic, it is a good idea to ask whether or not the patient has had any previous adverse reactions.

• Bleeding. Reassure patients that major bleeding is very uncommon (they often fear it the most). However, it is a risk they should be aware of.

• Infection.

• Advise about the likelihood of waking up with drains from the wound, an O_2 mask and NGT. Drains and NGT may stay in place for several days. Advise also that post-op nausea from the anaesthetic is possible and that post-op pain will be treated.

Expected side effects after surgery

Amputation. Sloughing; cramps; phantom pain; psychological distress; need for revision.

Aortic aneurysm repair. Bleeding; thrombo-embolism; ureteric damage; paraplegia (from anterior spinal artery damage); gut ischaemia; ARDS; renal failure; aorto-enteric fistula. Also fatigue and feeling low. These patients usually go to ITU post-op.

Biliary surgery. Jaundice; strictures; pancreatitis; hepato-renal syndrome; bleeding. Drainage tubes in place.

Abdominal/colonic surgery. Constipation (ileus); fistulae; anastomotic leaks; obstruction; trauma to ureters. The patient will need counselling about a stoma; contact your stoma nurse to arrange this if the nurses have not already done so. Always consent patients undergoing colonic surgery for ileostomy/colostomy and warn them that they may have one when they wake up.

Cavity surgery. Sepsis. Ureteral and renal damage. Infection.

Mastectomy. Arm oedema; anxiety/depression.

Splenectomy. Infection (pneumococcal septicaemia); thrombocytosis. The patient should have been given pneumo-

coccal, HiB ± meningococcal vaccines at least 1 week prior to surgery; if not, they need it. Consult immediately with seniors. Splenectomized patients need prophylactic antibiotics (penicillin V 250–500 mg bd) probably for the rest of their lives (people have died of pneumococcal sepsis 20 years post-op). They will also need advice about coping with the side effects of antibiotics (diarrhoea, candidiasis, particularly vaginal thrush). They also need a card and preferably a medical bracelet to alert others that they have no spleen.

Thyroid surgery. Bleeding; hoarseness (laryngeal nerve palsy).

Tracheostomy. Stenosis; mediastinitis; surgical emphysema.

Prostatectomy. Urinary retention post-op; urethral stricture and incontinence; bleeding; retrograde ejaculation (usually asymptomatic but important to mention!).

Haemorrhoidectomy. Bleeding and anal stricture.

Anaesthetics

Make friends with your firm's anaes-thetist. Anaesthetists usually visit their patients (and you) the evening before theatre. Having everything ready for them saves a lot of headaches.
• Get an anaesthetic rota from the anaesthetic department. This saves telephone calls when you need to find the anaesthetist to warn them of late changes or patient complications.
• Tell your anaesthetist about (a) late

changes to a patient or procedure, (b) high risk patients.

• Check whether you or the anaesthetist need to prescribe the pre-medication.

• Arrange for ECGs to be done on admission for anyone older than 50.

• Arrange for CXRs to be done on patients well in time for theatre as local protocols require (routine pre-op CXRs are not recommended by the Royal College of Radiologists, see p. 180).

• Arrange for neck X-rays to be done on patients with rheumatoid arthritis.

• Write a checklist in the notes for patients going to theatre. The following is routine, but add or subtract lines depending on your specialty.

Pre-op checklist
Premed — prescribed/given.......
NBM for x hours...............
FBC:...........................
C&E:...........................
ECG — done/NA...............
CXR + report..................
(No) sickle cell disease, liver disease,
    COAD, CVS disease..........
(No) allergies.................
Special needs:.................

• Have the anaesthetist help you to insert cannulae if you have trouble. It is much less stressful putting them into unconscious patients.

• Ask the anaesthetist to teach you how to intubate patients.

Drawing up theatre lists

Some hospitals require House Officers to do this.

• Include: Name of the surgeon to do each case.
  Name of the theatre.
  Date and time the list is supposed to start.
  Name, sex, age, hospital number and ward of each patient.
  Procedure.
  Special information (for example, high risk status).

• Put children and diabetics first.

• Put 'dirty' (bowel) surgery and high risk patients last.

• Let theatre staff know that a patient is high risk so they can get prepared.

Marking patients for surgery

• Use an indelible pen and mark boldly.

• Discuss varicose vein marking with the surgeon.

Post-operative care

Post-op patients are usually much less work than pre-op patients. However, be alert to post-op emergencies as well as slow onset complications. PEs, stress-induced heart failure, MI, haemorrhage, anaesthetic and steroid reactions, as well as terrible pain all require urgent action. It is *vital* to remember emergency routines for these problems, even if you do not use them much during your surgical rotation. Nursing staff on surgical convalescent wards may not know much about medical emergencies and it may be up to you to start rapid treatment.

1 It is a good idea to conduct your own daily ward round, particularly if you are on call for the evening. Dunn and Rawlinson provide a useful ward round

checklist that enables you to take command of your ward:*
• Ask the patient about pain, breathing, eating, bowels and bladder output.
• Examine the chest, abdomen, wound, legs, mental state.
• Check drains, lines and catheters for drainage and local infection. Are they still necessary?
• Look at the charts for pyrexia, tachy-cardia and changes in BP and fluid balance.
• Make sure the patient is written up for adequate analgesia, night sedation, antibiotics and fluids. Are they all still necessary?
• Order investigations:
  • FBC, C&E post-op.
  • C&E daily for as long as the patient is on a drip.
  • Other tests to check for specific complications of different operations.
2 Remember to look for the '4W' com-plications: Wound, Walking, Wind, Water (i.e. wound infection, DVT, chest infection/PE and poor urine output). Ileus is also a common problem.

Complicated patients

Jaundice

Problems: excessive bleeding and dehy-dration, resulting in hepato-renal syn-drome if not treated, liver disease.
Do:
• Pre- and post-op liver function tests, INR and APTT.
• Avoid morphine in pre-medication.

* Dunn D.C. & Rawlinson N. (1999). *Surgical Diagnosis and Management: A Guide to General Surgical Care.* Blackwell Science, Oxford.

• Ensure adequate IV fluids. Hydrate pre-op if necessary (care if heart failure, ascites or low albumin). Use 5% dex-trose, not saline.
Consider:
• Pre-op vitamin K.
• Pre-op renal dose dopamine.
• Post-op 2-hourly urine output check.
• Post-op IV fluids to match fluid losses (urine, NGT, stool).
• Measure C&E daily.
• Avoid saline if the person is in liver failure and has ascites.

Diabetes

Problems: hypoglycaemia; ketoacidosis precipitated by stress and dehydration; post-op infection. Also, this group has a high percentage of silent MIs. For surgi-cal protocol see Table 15.2.

For all diabetics

• Consider ECG.
• Check local protocols.

For well-controlled NIDDM

• Do pre-op fasting glucose (preferably the day before surgery).
• If pre-op fasting glucose is less than 11 mmol/l, halve the oral hypoglycaemic dose the day before surgery and omit the oral hypoglycaemic on the day of surgery.
• If pre-op fasting glucose is greater than 11 mmol/l, follow the IDDM regime in Table 15.2.
• For minor procedures and even larger procedures if the patient is eating on the same day, simply omit the morning hy-poglycaemic. Institute IV insulin/GKI (Table 15.3) if uncontrolled (BM > 10).

Table 15.2 Surgical protocols for people with diabetes.

	Minor surgery (eating same day)	Major surgery, especially GI (not eating for several days)
Well-controlled NIDDM	• Omit morning hypoglycaemic drugs	• Omit hypoglycaemic drugs • Monitor blood glucose qds • GKI/sliding scale if insulin needed
Poorly controlled NIDDM and IDDM	• Omit morning insulin • Monitor blood glucose • Return to usual regime as soon as eating • NIDDM may need insulin on a PRN basis	• Keep on GKI/IV sliding scale/qds insulin until eating

Table 15.3 The GKI (Glucose, Potassium, Insulin) regime—as used in Newcastle.

500 ml of 10% dextrose with 10 mmol KCl and variable insulin, usually 12–16 units Actrapid. Infuse at 80 ml/hour

If blood glucose 7–10 continue
If blood glucose >10 and rising, put up a new bag containing 4 more units of insulin than previously
If blood glucose <7, use a new bag with 4 units *less* insulin
Blood glucose <3 give 200 ml 10% dextrose and re-check the blood glucose

The rationale of this regime is that it provides both insulin and dextrose. It thus suppresses ketone production and avoids problems that might occur with separate insulin and glucose infusions, such as the glucose drip finishing or blocking while the insulin drip carries on, potentially causing hypoglycaemia

• If the patient is undergoing major surgery, follow the GKI and omit the oral hypoglycaemic agent on the day of surgery.

For IDDM and poorly controlled NIDDM

• Put the patient first on the list and tell the surgeon (or theatre sister) that the patient is diabetic.
• Pre-op fasting glucose, urea, C&E, FBC (at least).
• Ensure good IV access pre-op (at least a green cannula).

• If the operation is in the morning, omit all insulin or hypoglycaemic drugs.
• Use the GKI regime (see Table 15.3).

Insulin infusion

• Draw up 50 units of short-acting insulin (for example, Actrapid) in a 50 ml syringe and then fill the syringe with 50 ml of normal saline. This means that there is 1 unit of insulin/ml, allowing easy adjustment according to the sliding scale shown in Table 15.4.
• Label the syringe.
• Set up an infusion pump (p. 102) or

Table 15.4 Insulin sliding scale.

Fingerprick glucose (mmol)	IV soluble insulin (units/hour)
<2	None. Give 50 ml of 50% glucose. Call doctor
4.0–6.4	0.5
6.5–8.9	1
9.0–10.9	2
11.0–16.9	3
17.0–28.0	4
>28	8 Call doctor

put the syringe in the fridge and let the nurses know where it is.

• To convert this scale to a SC scale, give four times the IV dose. This is because SC insulin is given every 4 hours instead of every hour.

• Work out how much insulin the patient normally receives, in whatever form. For example, if he or she gets a total of 100 units/24 hours as a mixture of long and short acting insulin, then adjust the sliding scale so that roughly 100 units of short acting insulin is given over 24 hours. However, you will need to reduce the normal dose while the patient is not eating.

• Make sure you check C&E at least once daily while the patient is on a sliding scale of insulin and a K infusion. Adjust K accordingly. Remember that K comes out of cells as blood glucose rises and can quickly drop once the patient's glucose comes under control.

• If the fingerprick glucose is persistently >11, increase each insulin dose on the sliding scale by 0.5–1.0 units. On the other hand, if the fingerprick glucose is constantly <4.0 mM reduce each insulin dose on the sliding scale by 0.5–1.0 units.

Steroid-dependent patients

(see The steroid patient, p. 115)

Problem: risk of life theatening hypotension (Addisonian crisis). Steroid-dependent patients need extra steroid cover for surgical stress.

• Ensure good IV access.

• Major surgery: give 100 mg hydrocortisone IM/IV with pre-med, then 6-hourly for 3 days.

• Minor surgery: as above, but only give post-op hydrocortisone for 24 hours.

Thyroid surgery

Problems: vocal chord damage, post-op thyroid storm, bleeding.

• Have vocal chords checked by ENT pre-op.

• Cross-match at least 2–4 units and G&S post-op.

• Ensure good IV access.

• Measure Ca post-op.

• Patients who have undergone thyroid surgery should have clip removers at the bedside. If they bleed suddenly the surgical clips should be removed to prevent suffocation and to allow the bleeding to be controlled directly with pressure.

Day surgery

More and more operations are being done as day surgery; the Royal College of Surgeons' target is 50%.
• Don't spend too much time clerking day surgery patients (usually 5–10 minutes). They have usually been checked over at least twice already. However, you do need to ensure they have no obvious CVS or respiratory problems (like a recent cold), and if necessary, to send them home.
• Develop a protocol clerking sheet for your day patients (see p. 187).
• Prescribe adequate take-home analgesia. Poor pain relief is the most common problem for patients—and for GPs who have to prescribe it.* A few paracetamol are not adequate postoperatively. Co-proxamol (2 tabs) 4–6-hourly is standard, but check with your surgeons and the nursing staff.
• Tell patients what to expect, especially within the first 24 hours. For instance, fatigue and wound-related discomfort are normal. Tell patients that you are giving them pain killers to take home with them and that they should use them!
• Tell patients:
    They can't drive for 48 hours and they certainly can't drive home.
    They can eat and drink.
    They should have a contact number for the hospital and their GP should any problems arise (it is helpful to give the hospital day surgery contact number to patients and their relatives).
• Your senior is responsible for discharging patients from day surgery. Legally you are not supposed to sign discharge forms for patients until you have full medical registration.

Oro-facio-maxillary surgery

Being a House Officer for the oro-facio-maxillary surgeons usually involves rapid clerking of patients who are going to have their teeth pulled, usually their wisdom teeth. These patients are often teenagers and rarely present problems:
• Make sure you get under-16 parental consent while the parents are on ward, otherwise you will have to bring them in from home to sign the consent form.
• Try writing and photocopying a prototype clerking sheet for these patients.
• Always ask about heart lesions and blood clotting disorders. Listen for murmurs. Have a list of antibiotics for prophylactic cover in your filofax or folder to fill into the drug chart.
• Know how to read dental shorthand for teeth:
(European version)
Adults

R $\dfrac{8+7+6+5+4+3+2+1+|+1+2+3+4+5+6+7+8}{8-7-6-5-4-3-2-1-|-1-2-3-4-5-6-7-8}$ **L**

Children

R $\dfrac{5+4+3+2+1+|+1+2+3+4+5}{5-4-3-2-1-|-1-2-3-4-5}$ **L**

• Examples of teeth notation:
    The upper and lower right wisdom teeth is $\underline{8}+/\overline{8}-$
    The upper left wisdom tooth is $+\underline{8}$
    The lower left wisdom tooth is $-\overline{8}$

* Dr Jean Miller. Day Surgery Workshop. Sponsored by Anglia and Oxford Regional Health Authority, 15 June 1994.

- Take to the bedside:
  Blood cards and bottles for FBC, U&E, INR.
  Clerking sheet.
  Drug chart.
  Consent form.
  Stethoscope.

Surgical protocol clerking sheet

Figure 15.1 is a condensed example of a surgical protocol clerking sheet that you might want to reproduce to ensure comprehensive, legible clerking. You may need to modify it to suit your particular specialty. It is also a good idea to leave plenty of space for additional comments for patients whose details are not covered by the protocol.

It is easy to photocopy the protocol directly onto your hospital's clerking forms, but you first need to make a template to photocopy from. Place a clerking form beneath some plain A4 paper and scroll both into a typewriter so that the plain paper is on top. Type out the first page of the protocol onto the plain paper so that it lines up with underlying form. Repeat for the second (and maybe third) page of the protocol. Alternatively you can use a word processor and adjust the page margins to fit the hospital forms. Load a photocopier's tray with hospital forms and photocopy the protocol onto them.

Chapter 16: **Self care**

How doctors are supposed to take care of patients without resentment if they don't take care of themselves is beyond us. Most are not taught much about self care in medical school. Look after yourself and become a more humane doctor in the process.

Accommodation

Although in practice no-one checks to see that you are living on-site, hospitals have a duty to provide acceptable accommodation without charge. National regulations governing minimum acceptable standard which hospitals are obliged to comply with include:

• Your room should contain a 3-by-6 foot bed, telephone, cupboards, drawers, desk, chair, armchair, washbasin, be carpeted and have curtains. It should be heated and regularly cleaned.

• There should be a nearby bathroom and toilet, cooking facilities, a common room and on-site laundry facilities. Common areas should be regularly cleaned.

• On-call rooms should have clean sheets, a phone and a clean room. Call the Domestic Supervisor if there is a problem.

If you have a specific problem with your quarters, contact the designated 'Accommodation officer' or equivalent through switchboard. This person will also supply you with replacement light bulbs, toilet paper, etc. If the quarters *en bloc* are below standard, involve your doctors' mess and the junior doctors' committee.

Alternative careers

What if you have come all this way and you find that you don't want to be a doctor? Or you like it, but not enough to dedicate your life to it? Little known to many medics, having a medical degree opens many great doors. Chekhov, Maugham, Florey and Keats were all once doctors—to name a few.

• Medical training gives you all sorts of skills that you probably never even noticed. These include interviewing, analytic, mechanical, adversarial, communicating and observational skills, the ability to work within a hierarchy and still get what you want, sheer endurance and persistence (much prized in the workforce), experience of the human condition at its most vulnerable—and many others. Never think that these are wasted in a 'non-medical' career. Having medical training will enable you to bring something special to whatever you do.

• Having said that, *in general* we would advise doing at least your house job before saying good-bye to medicine. Many people find that they enjoy working much more than being a student. Without the house job year, it is hard to assess what it is all about. In any case, having full registration is useful if you ever wish to work in the future.

Bleep

• Pick up your bleep from switchboard. They will replace the batteries.
• If your bleep is too loud, cover the speaker with masking tape.
• If your bleep switches off too easily, tape can also be used to prevent the switch from moving.
• Leave your bleep on the ward (or switch it off) if you are not on-call, as switchboard may call you even when you are off-duty.

British Medical Association (BMA)

Becoming a member of the BMA not only brings you the *BMJ* with all the job adverts for next year, but provides advice and support in all areas of your work, leave, contracts, tax and financial planning. It is also of national importance as a negotiating body on behalf of all doctors. While the New Deal for Junior Doctors is not perfect, it nonetheless has been a major step forward in improving junior doctors' hours and re-defining appropriate duties for House Officers. Specific benefits of membership include.

1 Personal advice on contracts and terms of service.
2 Assistance and representation in disagreements with hospital management. This is becoming more important as Trusts and management try to change contracts and reduce pay. For example, the BMA has threatened court action against trust management which has tried to cut pay, now protected under the New Deal terms. The BMA can assist with claims for overtime and additional hours.
3 Independent financial advice by salaried representatives on pensions, income protection, etc.
4 Insurance services. The personal contents policy is particularly useful .
5 The fee is tax deductible.

Car and insurance

You may buy your first car during your house job year. While you may need to purchase in July just prior to moving to your new job, cars are most expensive around July–August. Also, your hospital is obliged to reimburse you for moving expenses, so you do not necessarily need your own car to move.

Car insurance varies a lot. The BMA offers insurance for doctors, but it may be more expensive than you need if you have bought an old car. Probably the best thing to do is to ring local brokers who deal with many different insurance firms and who can get you the best deal for the cover you need. Many firms give a discount for young female drivers. Be aware that you can purchase third party insurance ± fire and theft, if your car is not valuable.

Clothes (laundry/stains)

• Find out how to exchange white coats. A clean coat helps your morale and professional demeanour, although it is *not* more hygienic.

- Remove blood from washable items by soaking them in warm (not hot), soapy water with added salt and then washing them regularly. Sponging the item as soon as possible helps too. For old stains, soak or wash the item in a soapy solution containing a few drops of ammonia or hydrogen peroxide.
- Remove blood from non-washable items by sponging with cold water. Cover silk with a paste of starch and water; allow to dry and brush off.
- Alternatively, *Stain Devils* remove most stains. You can buy them in large supermarkets or at dry-cleaning outlets. Make sure you buy the right one for the stain you have. *Stain Devils* are particularly useful for ink and ball-point stains.
- Finally, most stains can be removed with dry-cleaning. Hospitals should reimburse you for dry cleaning costs if you got the stain at work. Contact Personnel through the switchboard to find out how to apply for reimbursement.

Contacting medical colleagues

After graduation, all doctors are entered into the UK Medical Directory. This is a reasonably reliable way of tracking down friends from medical school and beyond. The Directory is available in hospital libraries and also from the General Medical Council nearest you. There are now Internet services dedicated to doctors, which provide a lifelong email address for all subscribers, and can supply doctors with contact details of colleagues who have also subscribed.

Contract and conditions of service

Doctors' working conditions are negotiated by the Junior Doctors' Committee. More recently, the Junior Doctors' New Deal agreement has altered the rates at which overtime is paid, and stipulated the maximum hours for which you can be contracted to work. All hospitals, including Trusts, have to abide by these nationally agreed guidelines.

What you need to know about your contract

Your contract is a binding agreement, regulating your hours and conditions of service, pay, holiday and notice. It cannot be altered unilaterally by either you or your employer. In particular, under the Junior Doctors' New Deal, your pay cannot be cut, even if the hours of work are reduced. The pay and hours system has been recently reviewed. Contact your local BMA office or go on-line at www.bma.org.uk for full details.

1 Rota

Most House Officers still work a basic on-call rota (e.g. 1 in 5), meaning that they work a 40-hour working week and are also on duty every fifth night and every fifth weekend. Partial and full shifts refer to the workload during your period of work and not to the timetabling. They do stipulate the maximum number of hours you work and the amount of time you must have off. Prospective cover means that when colleagues are away on holiday, the remaining House Officers cover the nights the

Table 16.1 New Deal hours.

Rotation pattern	Maximum continuous work	Minimum period off duty between work periods	Minimum continuous period off duty
Full shift	14 hours	8 hours	48 hours + 62 hours in 28 days
Partial shift	16 hours (except 24 hour partial shifts)	8 hours	48 hours + 62 hours in 28 days
On-call rota	32 hours (56 hours at weekend)	12 hours	48 hours + 62 hours in 21 days

missing colleague would have done. This works out equitably if everyone takes the same amount of holiday. Virtually all contracts stipulate that you cover your colleagues if they are sick. This provision does *not* give authorities power to force you to cover foreseen and notified absences such as annual leave. The New Deal stipulates a maximum of 72 working hours per week for on-call rotas, 64 hours for partial shift and 56 hours for full shift, and applies controls to these hours as shown in Table 16.1.

2 Pay

NHS doctors' rates of pay are agreed nationally by the Doctors and Dentists' Review Body, which negotiates the annual pay increase each April. Your pay is calculated on the basis of a banding system. The banding system takes into consideration the type of rota worked and the duration and intensity of out of hours work. Your band dictates the supplement received over basic salary. House officers in General Practice who have an out-of-hours commitment receive an additional 22.5% over and above basic salary regardless of the duration or frequency of that commitment. The BMA website (bma.org.uk) features a band calculator, allowing you to check that your employer is complying with New Deal requirements. At the time of writing, pay ranges from £21 522 (band 1c) to £29 055 (band 3).

• Your band is specified in your contract. The band allocation should take into account prospective cover and expected early starts and late finishes, such as 8 am ward rounds.

Overtime for early starts and late finishes can (in theory) be paid retrospectively. It requires your consultant to sign the appropriate claim form, confirming your extra work. In practice it can be difficult to achieve. Consultants and management may not look kindly on such claims, although this varies considerably from hospital to hospital.

• While the odd hour here or there probably does not warrant special overtime claims, if you are systematically working extra hours (for example, by starting at 8 am instead of 9 and finishing at 7 pm instead of 5), then do not feel ashamed of asking for pay for honest work that you have done.

• *Always* document exactly (to the

minute) when you start and finish work on a special 'overtime' sheet in your folder or filofax. Documentation substantially reinforces pay claims.

3 Holiday

House Officers are entitled to 5 weeks holiday/year, or two and a half weeks/6 month job, excluding Bank holidays.
• Try to avoid carrying leave forward. In theory, up to 4 days leave can be carried forward from the first job to the second, but this is often hard to achieve. Contact Personnel both at your current hospital and your future place of work to try to ensure you are granted the extra leave.
• Leave can be supplemented by 'in-lieu' days. Over the year you are likely to work several bank holidays and statutory hospital holidays. You can take a day off 'in-lieu' of each holiday worked or if you work over-night beyond 9 am on the holiday morning.
• Find out the procedure for booking leave early. It may involve simply informing your consultant and his or her secretary, or there may be specific forms to be filled in and signed by your consultant.

4 Notice

House Officers only need to give 2 weeks notice of their intention to leave their post. However, to be eligible for full GMC registration you need to have completed 10 months as an House Officer, including 4 months of medicine and 4 months of surgery. It is not unheard of for House Officers to be given notice if the employing hospital is cutting back staff. In this unfortunate circumstance you will simply have to look for another job. However, there are often good job vacancies at short notice. Talk to the dean's office of your medical school and look in the *BMJ Classifieds* that come every week with the non-student version of the *BMJ*.

5 Leave

Compassionate leave

In the event of family or personal bereavement, paid leave will usually be given. Tell your consultant. If there is any difficulty, talk to your clinical tutor and Personnel.

Maternity (and paternity) leave

Regulations and rates of parental leave are complex, depending on how long you have worked and whether you intend to return to work. Female House Officers are unlikely to have worked for more than 1 year and, therefore, are allowed only 18 weeks unpaid leave. By comparison, doctors who have worked for longer than 1 year are entitled to 8 weeks full pay, 10 weeks half pay and up to 34 weeks of additional leave, to a total absence of 52 weeks. Doctors who have not declared intention to return to work receive fewer benefits.
• If you or your partner is pregnant or considering it, discuss the options for leave fully with your personnel department or the BMA.
• Sadly, unlike the rest of the European Union, the UK does not yet have paid paternity leave as an entitlement for employees. However, if you are an expectant father and need time off, it is worth discussing with your employer and the BMA.

Study leave

Pre-registration doctors are not allocated study leave other than time during the working day to attend clinical and pathology meetings. Post-registration doctors are entitled to 30 days of study leave per year.

Sick leave

Physical illness. It is still the case in most hospitals that if you are sick, your colleagues must cover you in addition to doing their own jobs. Because of this very few doctors will tell you to go home. Therefore, you *must* take control of the situation and go home if you need to. You may not be on death's door, but if you are struggling to keep up with your tasks *just go home*. The ward will cope. They might even celebrate. You are doing nobody any favours by lurking around shedding your virus and bad temper.

Mental illness. If you are struggling with mental burn out (depression, serious anxiety, grief, whatever) it is more important that you do some self diagnosis and get help and rest. Mental fatigue and illness is so common amongst doctors yet so little spoken about. It is also a cause of long-term absence and loss of self esteem which could be avoided with a bit of self care.

If you have trouble with illness of any kind, consider doing the following:
• Tell someone who loves you that you're sick/in trouble. They can help you summon up the courage to take time off and get help.
• See the hospital staff's doctor or nurse

or your GP. They can help you medically and psychologically. They will give you any documentation you need (e.g. sick notes) and may be able to speak with your seniors if necessary. You are obliged to tell your consultant that you're sick (after 3 days absence). Unlike more junior colleagues, your consultant won't suffer directly if you take time off and will probably be sympathetic.
• Tell your immediate senior and the nurses on your wards so they can make arrangements for cover as soon as possible.
• Learn to care for yourself now and it will serve you throughout your life. This is preferable to a heart attack or Chronic Martyrdom Syndrome when you're 45.

Prolonged illness

Even if you fall ill on the first day of work and cannot work again, you are still entitled to sick pay equal to your full salary for 1 month. After this you will receive the usual state benefits. After completing 4 months full time work, an House Officer is entitled to 1 month of full pay and 2 months of half pay. If you fall ill towards the end of the contract and the illness continues after the time when you would have finished, you are entitled to continued sick pay as long as the illness lasts or until you have had all the sick pay you are entitled to.

6 Occupational health requirements

• Hospitals recommend that you register with a local GP, although in practice your notes will barely have caught up with you when you have to move on.
• On arrival at the hospital, the Occupa-

tional Health Department will ask about your immunization record. They may take nose or other swabs, particularly if you have worked in a different region or where there has been an MRSA (methicillin resistant *Staphylococcus aureus*) outbreak.

• Ask Occupational Health to check your Hep B immunity which may have dramatically declined since immunization as a student. It should be approximately '100%'. If you do become infected with Hep B you cannot be a surgeon or a specialist who does invasive work. See below for needlestick injuries.

• Contact the Occupational Health Department if you are ill for longer than 3 days. They will clear you for sick leave and may well give you some TLC in the meantime.

Doctors' mess

The doctors' mess may be a scruffy room strewn with old newspapers and coffee cups or a comfortable lounge with a coffee machine, satellite TV and a PlayStation. Most messes run with a Mess President, Secretary and Treasurer and a variable number of committee members. If there is not much going on, organize an event and take command!

Making money for the mess

• Have regular drug lunches and charge the reps £100 to talk while you provide the catering at £50 per session.

• Organize with your colleagues and the financial people handling cremation fees for a part of each cremation fee to be given to the mess (e.g. £3).

• Hold a party. Have free drinks before

8.30 pm to make sure everyone arrives early, or no-one will come until the pubs close.

• Ask doctors to make a regular deduction from their salary and arrange this with Personnel.

Drug representatives

Drug company representatives will approach you from time to time to try to influence your prescribing policy. You need to decide for yourself how you deal with them and their practice of bribing doctors with items and services (ranging from pens to dinners at local restaurants). Just a few tips:

• You are not obliged to spend time with drug reps. You can tell them politely that you do not have time to see them, or that you are not interested in discussing their products.

• On the other hand, you can influence drug availability by talking with company representatives. For instance, you can point out that such-and-such antibiotic would be more practical if it could be made up in solution and left in the fridge (like metronidazole) for a few hours, rather than needing to be given stat.

• Be wary of drug company literature. While some is reliable, much of it is misleading. To learn about drugs you'd be better off reading a pharmacology textbook, the *BNF* or the *Drug and Therapeutics Bulletin* which you receive free as an House Officer.

Insurance (room contents)

Probably the best room contents insurance against theft and damage is BMA-arranged insurance, because it is designed specifically for junior doctors. Other policies may not have plans appropriate for your unusual living situation and generally cost much more.

Jobs

• Your SHO post is where the big divide begins: surgery/medicine/general practice. If you're not sure (most people aren't), 6 months of A&E is useful. Otherwise choose a general rotation. Ask your consultants, friends and older colleagues where the good jobs are.
• Network. Tell your consultant what you're hoping to do next. If you are set on a particular job or hospital, ask the consultant if he or she knows anyone there. A quick consultant-to-consultant chat is a time honoured way of securing the next post.
• Choose your referees carefully. One is usually the consultant you are currently working for. Well known professors and consultants add a little weight to your list—provided you actually know them well enough for them to write about you, and you are sure that they will say nice things!
• Application form. Make sure you get the basics right. If it asks to be typed or printed in green ink, do it. Include photographs or whatever else is requested. Don't jeopardize your chances at this early stage. Consider using recorded or registered delivery.

Curriculum vitae

It is probably easiest to type out your CV yourself so you can make small changes as necessary. Use high quality paper. Your consultant's secretary might oblige.
• Make sure you spell-check your CV—or proof read it carefully for misspellings. Read your CV aloud to make sure that it does not contain any disastrous sentences or factual errors.
• Try to be concrete about what you want to do. People love hearing concrete plans that are easy for them to imagine. If you know what your planned career is, say so. Put 'Career objective: chest medicine' at the top of your CV under your name.
• Make the most of your experience, listing skills you have acquired and responsibilities you have taken. Don't forget skills such as computing and languages. Make sure you include honours or prizes, even from school.
• Avoid one-word interests such as 'Reading'. Try to be concrete in demonstrating what you have done. For example, instead of saying 'Running', you might specify your running activities: 'Participation in Anglia regional running events, club secretary'.
• Create your CV so it shows you as you want to be seen. CVs are not shopping lists, nor are they confessions. If you did badly one year you can minimize the fact in how you present your CV. Just make sure that you don't say things that are blatantly untrue, and that you include certain professional details (see later).
• When asking for a reference, supply your referee with a current CV and brief outline of achievements you want them to mention.
• Show your CV to your Mum or a close friend to make sure that you haven't left anything important out. Consider showing it to your present

colleagues/consultant and secretaries who have probably seen many CVs and can give you good advice on both content and style.

• If the form you are given for your CV is inadequate, staple your CV to it, unless the instructions strictly state otherwise.

A CV should include (at least):

Personal: name, address, nationality, date of birth, civil status, interests, brief general education, and non-medical employment (if any).

Medical: undergraduate education including medical school, date of entry and graduation, honours or prizes, qualifications, previous and present appointments, career plans, publications, society memberships, referee names and telephone and fax numbers.

The interview

• Try to visit the hospital before the interview, see the department and meet the consultants. If you have already met some of the interview panel you may be more relaxed.

• Follow the basics: clean suit, hair and shoes, be punctual and courteous.

• Find out from the person coordinating the interview what you can expect inside the interview room, such as how many interviewers you will face and the expected length of the interview.

• Early questions are likely to focus on your CV and experience. Be prepared to discuss and expand on anything you have mentioned. At this level it is rare that you will be asked medical questions. Be prepared for questions about your career plans. Try to say something concrete, even if you are unsure about your future

career. At all costs avoid looking aimless. Ethical issues such as euthanasia may be discussed. Issues such as quality control, audit and clinical governance are also likely to arise.

• Listen attentively to the interviewers' questions and take care to answer them directly rather than blurring the issue. Don't ramble.

• While remaining relatively formal, don't be afraid to be yourself. If the interviewer doesn't like you as you really are, you probably don't want to work for them anyway.

• Write thank you letters to your referees for their help and support. You may need them again in the future!

Consultant career prospects

The medical and dental staffing prospects are published annually in the journal *Health Trends*, published by the Department of Health. The prospects include the current number of SpRs, consultants, likely consultant vacancies and future consultant numbers, by specialty. The journal should be in your medical library; if not, ring the Department of Health in London.

Locums

Locums pay well if you can bear working through your holidays and weekends.

• Get registered with one or more locum agencies. These are advertised in the *BMJ Classifieds*. Medical personnel at your hospital will know the name of local agencies. Note that different agencies pay very different rates. Shop around.

• Try to negotiate travel expenses with the agency.

• If you secure a locum at a hospital you

don't know, the following is a checklist of things to do when you arrive:

1 Sign in at the switchboard. Sign-in registers what time you arrive at the hospital—the locum agency may check when working out your pay.

2 From switchboard and reception, pick up: bleep, keys, map of the hospital, identification (if necessary) and essential telephone numbers:
  • A&E.
  • Admissions.
  • Biochemistry (and on-call bleep number).
  • Haematology (and on-call bleep number).
  • Porters.
  • Wards.
  • Radiology department (and on-call bleep number).

3 Find out (on the hospital map) where these are:
  • Blood gas machines.
  • Canteen.
  • Doctors' residence.
  • Drinks machine.
  • ITU.
  • Radiology department.
  • Wards.

4 Bleep your senior and arrange to meet.

5 Dump your overnight bag in the doctors' residence.

6 Go to the wards and introduce yourself.

7 On the wards, stuff a folder (see p. 8) with: blood forms, history sheets, consents, fluid charts, drug charts, X-ray forms. Clip the phone numbers to the front of the folder.

8 Locate IV equipment, catheters, drug cupboard, resuscitation equipment.

9 Find out:

• Who gives IV drugs.
• If there is a phlebotomist in the morning and where to leave requests.

10 If possible, speak to the person who usually carries your bleep about any useful information he or she may know about patients, staff and the hospital.

11 If you are required to attend a ward round when you should have finished the locum, you are entitled to extra hours' pay; contact the locum agency as soon as possible about this. If you have to leave on the dot, let your senior know this from the outset.

12 Hospitals that are desperate to fill locums will often negotiate terms with you, such as allowing you to arrive late or leave early if necessary.

Meals

• Try not to miss meals. Twenty minutes for a hot evening meal makes little difference to patient care, but it will keep *you* going.

• Don't forget to drink as much liquid as possible. It's easy to get dehydrated and even more tired when you're too busy to stop for tea-breaks.

• If canteen food is awful, take in microwave meals. It's comforting to have a treat such as fruit or a chocolate bar.

• Find out about local take-aways. Some may discount hospital staff. There are almost always people on the shift who will share a meal with you and cut down the delivery cost.

Medical defence

Historically, it was compulsory to belong to a defence organization for representation and insurance against medicolegal complaints arising out of the care of patients. This changed in 1990 when Crown Indemnity came into force, so that the Crown, or rather the NHS employer, will pay the costs of investigation and damages for cases arising during your employment with them. However, protection under Crown Indemnity is limited. It does *not* cover incidents arising outside the hospital, such as 'good Samaritan' acts, nor private practice. Most importantly, Crown Indemnity may not support you if you have a conflict with your employer. The advantages of joining a medical defence organization are expert, round-the-clock advice with *your* interests at heart. Investigate the benefits offered by various organizations (e.g. MDU, MPS) and join whichever one suits your needs.

Money

For the first time, your bank account will be filling up with a £1250 or so each month. Be a bit careful. It's not unusual for people to run up thousands of pounds of credit card debts—and to spend the next few years paying them off.

Income protection if long-term sick or disabled

Various organizations offer income protection (also known as PHI or Permanent Health Insurance). On payment of a monthly premium, you are covered for prolonged absence, even if you never work again. If you have a mortgage and family, sickness cover becomes more im-

portant. Research the various policy options carefully.

Payslip deductions

National Insurance is a compulsory contribution which will pay for your future state pension, maternity pay and sick leave.

Superannuation is not compulsory but is essential for your pension. The national state pension is meagre. The NHS superannuation scheme is your employer's scheme to allow you to make additional pension contributions. You contribute 6% and the NHS contributes a further 4% of your basic salary (before tax and ADH additions).
• You have to sign a form at the start of your job stating your intention to stay with or opt out of the superannuation scheme. The only people who might not want to contribute towards their own superannuation are those who are pretty sure that they will not be working for long in the NHS, such as foreign graduates. However, NHS superannuation can be accrued to other public sector positions in the UK such as the civil service and university posts.
• You can reclaim superannuation contributions if you have worked for the NHS for *less than 2 years*. Otherwise your contributions will stay locked in the scheme.
• Think long and hard before leaving the superannuation scheme to join a private pension plan. It is highly unlikely that you could ever match the security and returns of the NHS scheme.

Pensions

As described above, the superannuation scheme provides the main pension for doctors. When you retire, your benefits are an annual pension of up to half your salary and a lump sum of three times your annual pension. The exact calculations are:

Pension = years of service/40 × pensionable salary

Pensionable salary = highest annual salary earned in any of the 3 years prior to retirement

• Few doctors complete the full 40 years of service that would allow them to receive the maximum possible pension. However, it is possible to make additional contributions to your future pension. The most cost-effective way is to make Additional Voluntary Contributions (AVCs) into the NHS Group Scheme. This is a well-kept secret, with low commission and charges. You should contact your local BMA office. It is also possible to buy 'added years', as if you had worked for longer than you really have.

• You will doubtless meet financial [illegible] [illegible] Standing AVCs, i.e. a way of investing your contributions in their company's policies (and earning them a bonus). Be aware that your whole first year's contribution may disappear in the salesperson's commission.

• Your expenses as a young doctor may be high—with a new house, a car and possibly a family. As long as you are aware that you should consider further pension contributions at some date, these need not be a priority in your first year of work (whatever financial advisers may say).

Tax

Earning a regular salary unfortunately means paying serious tax. You will save time, trouble and money if you make an effort to keep basic records. Each month you should get a payslip giving details of your pay, national insurance, and any other deductions you have authorized such as telephone bills or car parking charges. Check this to see you have not been overcharged.

A P60 is sent to you at the end of the tax year (5 April). It is your record of how much income you have received and tax you have paid. A P45 is given to you when you leave the job, to take to the finance department at your next job to show how much tax you have been paying. If you lose it you will probably be taxed the wrong amount (usually overtaxed) until the tax office sorts it out—which may take months.

Understanding your tax

Doctors have tax deducted automatically [illegible] [illegible] (known as PAYE—Pay As You Earn). The Inland Revenue works out how much tax you are likely to owe throughout the year and this is deducted monthly from your salary.

House Officers start work in August, part way through the tax year which runs from 6 April to 5 April. This means that your first pay cheque will be larger than any of the subsequent months. The tax year ends on 5 April. After this your tax office will send you a note stating how much tax you paid in the last year, and how much tax you ought to pay in the next year (P60). You could just leave it there. However, it is quite likely that you have been overtaxed and could claim money back on tax deductible items. You also have a duty to declare untaxed income so that it can be taxed. At the simplest, you could just write a letter declaring your tax deductible items and untaxed income; alternatively contact your tax office for a full tax return form. Your personnel department will be able to give you full details of your tax office, which is usually determined by where you work.

Tax deductible items (on which you can reclaim money you have paid in tax) include:

1 GMC fee (but only the renewal fee, not the initial joining-up fee).

2 Medical defence subscription.

3 BMA membership.

4 Replacement of medical equipment (e.g. better stethoscope).

5 Medical journals.

6 New books to replace old editions.

In later years, membership to one of the Royal Colleges is also tax deductible.

Untaxed income that must be declared

The main item here is cremation fees ('ash cash'), worth approximately £40, which you receive for completing part 1 of the cremation form. In recent years the Inland Revenue has tightened up on this potential evasion. It is not unknown for them to investigate funeral directors' records and compare them with doctors' tax returns. Non-declaration constitutes tax evasion and is penalized accordingly. You should declare full cremation fees even if there is a deduction, for example for mess expenses. Other untaxed cash payments such as the fees for completing other forms should also be declared.

Tax allowances

Everyone has a personal allowance, i.e. an amount of income they can earn before being taxed. In **2001/2** you earn £4535 (£5365 if you are married) before paying tax. The next £1880 is taxed at 10%; the next £27500 is taxed at 20%. The highest rate of 40% is paid on any income above this. This will not apply to House Officers unless you have substantial additional income.

Tax free savings

Each person is allowed to save up to £7000 each tax year in a tax-free savings account called an ISA (individual savings account). These accounts give high rates of tax-free interest, and are offered by most banks. There are various types of ISA on offer. Some (called 'cash' ISAs) guarantee growth of your savings (in effect a straight-forward tax-free savings account). Alternatively, you may choose an ISA where the bank will invest in named stocks and shares on your behalf. These 'equity' ISAs are more risky, especially if you may need to withdraw the money in the short term, but may have much greater yield in the longer term, although they can't guarantee that you will get back everything that you put in. ISAs seldom have instant access, so don't use them instead of a current account. However, they are a good way of putting away savings for the future. Seek financial advice to help you choose between the ISA packages on offer.

Telephone and on-line banking

Consider switching to telephone or on-line banking, which allow 24 hour access to your account, in addition to all the other services provided by a high street account (including use of cash machines). *Which?* magazine regularly reviews banking services so look out for the next *Which?* report. These accounts can offer a high rate of interest, although many exclusively on-line banks will offer these rates only as a promotion, with interest rates quickly falling back to more moderate (although often competitive) levels. Check to see that the on-line and other services offered fit your needs. Also be aware that exclusively on-line banks may not be covered by the banking ombudsman [the government watchdog for banks]. High street banks with on-line 'branches' are covered.

Needlestick injuries

If you needlestick yourself, do the following:
1 Squeeze blood from the site immediately. Go to a sink. Continue to squeeze blood from the wound under fast running, warm water.
2 See your occupational health consultant immediately (and inform your own consultant). You may need to take post-exposure anti-HIV prophylaxis (at present this consists of triple therapy).

3 Don't panic. Virtually all doctors needlestick themselves from time to time and very, very few have contracted anything undesirable, even from patients infected with HIV and hepatitis.
4 If they consent to it and are counselled about the implications of having an HIV test done, take one clotted (brown) tube of blood from the patient. This needs to be analysed immediately for HIV and hepatitis.
5 Alert your senior and/or the public health unit in the hospital. They will instruct you further. They will require you to do the following, depending on patient status.

If the patient is known to be HIV-positive

Don't panic. Thousands of HIV needlestick injuries have resulted in only a handful of cases of HIV worldwide. The chances of your getting HIV are very small. On the other hand, don't give yourself a hard time if you do panic. Almost everyone does, and people who haven't stuck themselves with HIV infected blood just don't understand what this is like. Seek help from a counsellor or GP if you are suffering from excessive anxiety about it.

1 Have one clotted tube of blood taken from yourself. Give it to the public health unit (GP for students). This is to ascertain your hepatitis/HIV status at the time of injury. It will only be analysed in the unlikely event that you are later found to be positive.
2 You will need to take anti-retroviral triple therapy for post-exposure prophylaxis. Seek the advice of your occupational health service.
4 After 3 months (at least) have an HIV

check. Over 95% of people who are going to seroconvert do so within 3 months. If this is negative, repeat it at 6 months and 1–2 years. The second test will give you peace of mind.

5 Use condoms at least until the 3 month check.

6 Having HIV tests does not usually pose a problem for getting life insurance (as it once did) if you explain that you are a health professional having a routine HIV check. However, if you are concerned, you can usually have your blood checked confidentially by your virology lab or the hospital's STD clinic (so it will not be recorded in your medical records). The latter is preferable, as you will get proper counselling for the test.

If the patient is known to be hepatitis-positive

1 Follow your doctor's instructions. Give the lab a clotted sample of your blood as soon as possible after injury to ascertain your hepatitis antibody status at the time of injury.

2 Find out what kind of hepatitis the patient has. They may have chronic hepatitis from lupus which is not infective. If they have Hep B, you may need instant immunoglobulin; if they have Hep C you may need interferon treatment.

3 You may need to be re-tested for hepatitis antigen after 6 months. In the meantime, it is advisable to practise safe sex.

Not coping

You are not alone. *Everyone* has disastrous days, weeks, months and even years. Everyone thinks about giving up medicine. If you feel like chucking it all in, this does not mean that you are less motivated or committed than anyone else. In fact the chances are that if you are feeling like that, so is everyone else, except that they'd rather die than admit it. Group studies suggest that when one person is feeling lonely, isolated, alienated and generally miserable, it is much more likely that others in the environment are too. Studies show that a substantial proportion of junior doctors become clinically depressed; most suffer depression and anxiety at least a few times during their career.

• Confidential counselling services have been established which provide counselling for doctors who are not coping. The BMA can advise you where such services are and how to contact them.

• Make sure that you do not blame yourself for structural problems in your workplace that have nothing to do with you. For instance, a bullying consultant or charge nurse will make anyone's life hell, not just yours. Consider talking to others—or even to your local BMA rep—about such problems, before taking it all upon yourself.

• Everyone experiences considerable turbulence upon entering the workplace. Remember that feeling low or anxious may just be manifestations of adjusting to a completely new way of life, and will pass within a few months, however painful they seem at present.

• Simple fatigue can greatly exacerbate mental distress. If you are feeling miserable, try going to bed really early on your nights off.

Part-time work (flexible training)

• It is now possible to be a part-time House Officer. At present part-time House Officer jobs are individually negotiated and created by postgraduate tutors. Part-time usually means half time, doing half the number of on-call nights. Unfortunately, the corollary of doing half time is that you must be an House Officer for 2 years instead of one.
• It is possible to continue flexible part-time training as an SHO, up to and including consultant level. At Registrar level and above, national recognition and approval for part-time training is required. At SHO level, simple agreement with the Postgraduate Dean suffices.
• It is increasingly common to spend part of the House Officer year in general practice.

Representation of junior doctors

You can get a great deal done if you and your colleagues work together on agreed goals. You can act as a body in several ways:

Doctors mess, mess president and committee. This may meet regularly or on an ad-hoc basis. It usually has several roles: organization of social events, representation of junior doctors' interests to management, administration of mess funds, rooms, etc.

Junior doctors' division. This is usually a hospital committee which meets every few months to discuss issues relevant to junior doctors. The main frustration for House Officer representatives is that you rarely work at the hospital long enough to see changes implemented.

New Deal committee. Hospitals should have convened this committee or something similar to consider and implement the issues arising from the Junior Doctors' New Deal, i.e. reducing doctors' hours and delegating inappropriate duties.

BMA. Junior doctors may stand as BMA representatives for local, regional and national committees. You should be allowed a reasonable amount of time off to attend to these activities. In practice it is usually doctors beyond the House Officer year who have the career stability to embark upon medical politics.

Sleep

Those who have not been sleep deprived cannot understand what it's like to be obsessed by the thought of sleep. Admittedly the situation has much improved since the 1980s. However, you can get very run down if you don't take care of yourself.
• If you've had little or no sleep the night before, a shower and breakfast go a long way to prevent the awful grey feeling of fatigue.
• Ask someone else to hold your bleep for a few hours. Have a nap at lunch time in an on-call room.
• After long shifts, go to bed, go directly to bed, do not pass Go, do not collect £200! You will be grateful the next morning.

• Another trick is to sleep in a side room while on call. This radically cuts down time getting up and travelling across car parks and long corridors to the ward, and rarely results in more calls. In the morning you only have to get up minutes before the ward round. Always strip your own sheets in the morning.

Appendix A: Useful tests, numbers and other information

Addresses

Diabetes UK (formerly The British Diabetic Association), 10 Queen Ann Street, London W1M 0DD (web: www.diabetes.org.uk, tel: 020-7323 1531)

British Medical Association (and *BMJ*), BMA House, Tavistock Square, London WC1H 9JP (web: www.bma.org.uk, tel: 020-7387 4499)

Central Public Health Lab, 61 Colindale Avenue, London NW9 5HT (web: http://www.phls.co.uk; tel: 020-8200 4400)

Communicable Disease Surveillance Centre (for notifying diseases), 61 Colindale Avenue, London NW9 5DF (web: http://www.phls.co.uk; tel: 020-8200 6868)

Disabled Living Foundation (for advice on equipment), 380–384 Harrow Road, London W9 2HU (web: http://www.dlf.org.uk; tel: 020-7289 6111)

Driving and Vehicle Licensing Authority (www.dvla.gov.uk)

General Medical Council, 178 Portland Street, London W1N 6JE (web: www.gmcuk.org, tel: 020-7580 7642)

Medical Defence Union, 230 Blackfriars Rd, London SE1 8PJ (web: http://www.themdu.com; tel: 020-7202 1500)

Medical and Dental Defence Union of Scotland, Mackintosh House, 120 Blythwood Street, Glasgow G2 4EH (web: http://www.mddus.com; tel: 0141-221 5858)

Medical Protection Society, 33 Cavendish Square, London W1G 0PS (http://www.mps.org.uk; tel: 020-7399 1300)

Medical Sickness Society, Colmore Circus, Birmingham B4 6AR (web: http://www.medical-sickness.co.uk; tel: 0808-100 1884)

Multiple Sclerosis Society, 372 Edgeware Rd, London NW2 6ND (web: http://www.mssociety.org.uk; tel: 020-8438 0700)

NHS Direct, www.nhsdirect.nhs.uk (Tel: 0845 4647)

Poisons Information

Belfast	028 9024 0503
Birmingham	0121 507 5588
	0121 507 5589
Cardiff	029 2070 9901
Dublin	00353 1 837 9964
	00353 1 837 9966
Edinburgh	0131 536 2300
London	020 7635 9191

Barthel score

The Barthel score helps you to assess quickly whether someone can manage at home. It is particularly useful at social rounds. A total score of 15 or more is 'good'.

Bathing
- 0 dependent
- 1 independent (bath and shower, in and out)

Bladder
- 0 incontinent or catheterized and unable to cope alone
- 1 occasional incontinence (1/day)
- 2 fully continent

Bowels
- 0 incontinent
- 1 occasional incontinence (1/week)
- 2 fully continent

Dressing
- 0 dependent
- 1 needs some help (e.g. with buttons, laces)
- 2 independent

Feeding
- 0 dependent
- 1 needs some help (e.g. with cutting)
- 2 independent (food within reach)

Grooming
- 0 dependent (hair, teeth, shaving)
- 1 independent

Mobility
- 0 immobile without help
- 1 independent with wheelchair (includes turning)
- 2 walks with one person assisting
- 3 independent

Stairs
- 0 dependent
- 1 needs assistance (physical, verbal, mechanical)
- 2 independent (up and down)

Toilet
- 0 dependent
- 1 needs some help
- 2 independent (transfer, wiping, dressing)

Transfer
- 0 unable (cannot balance to sit)
- 1 needs major assistance (2 people) but can sit
- 2 needs minor assistance (physical or verbal)
- 3 independent

Glasgow Coma Scale

Eyes open
- 4 spontaneously
- 3 to voice
- 2 to pain
- 1 none

Verbal response
- 5 oriented
- 4 confused
- 3 inappropriate words
- 2 incomprehensible words
- 1 none

Motor response
- 6 obeys command
- 5 localizes to pain
- 4 withdraws
- 3 flexes
- 2 extends
- 1 none

Total (out of 15)
Serious: ≤8
Moderate: 9–12
Mild: 13–15

Mental Health Act

1 Always get senior advice before using the Mental Health Act.
2 Section 4 states that for an emergency admission, the nearest relative *or* an approved Senior Nurse *or* a social worker *or* a doctor *as well as* the medical recommendation of one doctor who must have seen the patient within the previous 24

hours, can apply for 72 hours of compulsory admission on the grounds of:
- Urgent necessity.
- Mental disorder requiring hospital admission.
- Danger to him/herself or others.

3 Section 5(2) states that a patient already in hospital as a voluntary patient can be detained for 72 hours under the same conditions as Section 4, except that it only requires a single medical recommendation by the doctor in charge of the patient's care, *or* another doctor on the staff of the hospital who is nominated by the doctor in charge.

4 Sectioning a patient does not permit you to treat a concurrent physical condition unless it is life threatening.

Mini-mental test score

There are several versions of the mini-mental test score. This is one of them. It gives you a quick, ball park measure of someone's mental state. This can be very useful in casualty or in the middle of the night. Falstein's full mental test score is outlined in the *Oxford Handbook of Clinical Medicine*.

1 What month is it?
2 What year is it?
3 Where are you now?
4 Recall an address (have the person repeat this after you and then ask it from them at the end of the other questions).
5 Name three objects (e.g. pen, hand, watch).
6 What is your name?
7 Start of World War I (1914) or World War II (1939)?
8 Name of the current UK monarch.
9 Name of the Prime Minister.

10 Count backwards from 20 to 1 without an error.
- When giving the patient an address to recall, use one that you know so that *you* remember it. There is nothing more embarrassing than failing your own mini-mental test!
- Questions 7–9 are culturally specific. They can be substituted for questions the patient is likely to know.

Notifiable diseases

Doctors are legally required to report notifiable diseases to their local medical officer for environmental health. The microbiology department know who this is, as do people at the town hall. Alternatively you can contact the Communicable Disease Surveillance Centre: 61 Colindale Avenue, London NW9 5EQ (Tel: 020-8200 6868).

Recognized notifiable diseases are those listed below.

Acute encephalitis
Acute poliomyelitis
Anthrax
Cholera
Diphtheria
Dysentery
Food poisoning
Leptospirosis
Malaria
Measles
Meningitis:
   meningococcal
   pneumococcal
   haemophilus influenzae
   viral
   other specified
   unspecified
Meningococcal septicaemia (without meningitis)

Mumps
Ophthalmia neonatorum
Paratyphoid fever
Plague
Rabies
Relapsing fever
Rubella
Scarlet fever
Smallpox
Tetanus
Tuberculosis
Typhoid fever
Typhus fever
Viral haemorrhagic fever
Viral hepatitis:
   Hepatitis A
   Hepatitis B
   Hepatitis C
   other
Whooping cough
Yellow fever

Results

The following are normal ranges for results of tests. However, every lab is different; make sure that you use their values, particularly for unusual tests, which require local calibration of lab equipment.

Consider copying the results that are important for your job onto a single sheet, which you can stick at the back of a folder or filofax for easy reference.

Haematology

APTT (factors VIII, IX, XI, XII)	35–45 seconds
Eosinophils	0.04–0.44 (1–6%) $\times 10^9/l$
ESR female	(age + 10)/2
ESR male	(age)/2
FDPs	lab dependent
Hb (male)	13.5–18 g/dl
Hb (female)	11.5–16 g/dl
Lymphocytes	1.3–3.5 (20–45%) $\times 10^9/l$
MCV	76–96 fl
Monocytes	0.2–0.8 (2–10%) $\times 10^9/l$
Neutrophils	2–7.5 (40–75%) $\times 10^9/l$
Platelets	$150–400 \times 10^9/l$
Prothrombin (INR) (factors I, II, VII, X)	10–14 seconds (expressed as ratio versus control. Normal INR is 1.0)
RCC (female)	$3.9–5.6 \times 10^{12}/l$
RCC (male)	$4.5–6.5 \times 10^{12}/l$
Reticulocytes	0.8–2% (25–100 $\times 10^9/l$)
WCC	$4–11 \times 10^9/l$

Biochemistry

Acid phosphatase (prostate)*	0–1 IU/l
Acid phosphatase (total)*	1–5 IU/l
ACTH	3.3–15.4 pmol/l
ADH	0.9–4.6 pmol/l
Albumin	35–50 g/l
Aldosterone	100–500 pmol/l
Alk phos	30–300 IU/l
Alpha fetoprotein*	<10 IU/l
ALT	5–35 IU/l
Amylase	0–180 U
Angiotensin II	5–35 units
AST	5–35 IU/l
Bicarbonate	24–30 mmol/l
Bilirubin	3–17 mmol/l

* Clotted tube.

Ca (ionized)	1–1.25 mmol/l
Ca (total)	2.12–2.65 mmol/l
Chloride	95–105 mmol/l
Cholesterol	3.9–7.8 (>5 is high) mmol/l
Cortisol (am)	280–700 nmol/l
Cortisol (pm)	140–280 nmol/l
Creatine kinase (males)	25–195 IU/l
Creatine kinase (females)	25–170 IU/l
Creatinine	70–150 mmol/l
CSF glucose	>2/3 of plasma glucose
Ferritin	20–300 mmol/l
Folate	5–6.3 nmol/l
FSH	2–8 U/l
GGT (males)	11–51 IU
GGT (females)	7–33 IU
Glucose (fasting)	4–6 mmol/l
Glycosylated Hb*	6–8.5%
Haptoglobin	20–125 mmol/l
Iron (male)	14–31 mmol/l
Iron (female)	11–30 mmol/l
LDH	240–545 IU/l
Mg	0.75–0.15 mmol/l
Osmolality	278–305 mOsm/kg
PTH	<0.1–0.7 mg/l
Phosphate	0.8–1.45 mmol/l
Potassium	3.5–5.0 mmol/l
Prolactin (males)	<450 units
Prolactin (females)	<600 units
Protein (total)	60–80 g/l
Red cell folate*	0.36–1.44 mmol/l
Sodium	135–145 mmol/l
TSH	0.5–5.0 U/l
T_4	70–140 nmol/l
Thyroxine (free)	9–22 pmol/l
TIBC*	54–75 mmol/l
Triglyceride	0.55–1.9 mmol/l
T_3	1.2–3.0 nmol/l
Urea	2.5–6.7 mmol/l
Uric acid (males)	210–480 mmol/l
Uric acid (females)	150–390 mmol/l

Vitamin B_{12}	0.13–0.68 nmol/l or >150 ng/l

Arterial blood gases

pH	7.35–7.45
Pao_2	>10.6 kPa
$Paco_2$	4.7–6.0 kPa
Base excess	±2 mmol/l
Bicarbonate	22–26 mmol/l
Type 1 respiratory failure	Pao_2 <8, $Paco_2$ <6
Type 2 respiratory failure	Pao_2 <8; $Paco_2$ >6

Useful biochemical formulae

$$\text{Anion gap} = (Na + K) - (Cl + HCO_3)$$
$$= 4-17 \, mmol/l$$

• The anion gap is made up of ions such as phosphate, sulphate, lactate.
• It is high in any condition with reduced clearance or excess production of any unmeasured anions (e.g. DKA, lactic acidosis).
• It is low in hyperalbuminaemia, liver disease and paraproteinaemias.

Corrected calcium = reported total Ca $+ 0.2 \times (40 - \text{the actual albumin})$

Creatinine clearance (males)
$$\frac{1.23 \times (140 - age) \times wt(kg)}{creatinine}$$

Creatinine clearance (females)
$$\frac{1.04 \times (140 - age) \times wt(kg)}{creatinine}$$

* Clotted tube.

Fitness to drive

Condition	Normal licence	Notification of DVLC	Vocational licence
Anaesthetic	Avoid for 48 hours post-general anaesthetic	No	
Angina, chronic and stable	Avoid driving if symptomatic while driving	No	Many restrictions; refer to DVLC
Angioplasty	1 month	No	Check with DVLC
Aortic aneurysm	No restrictions	Yes	Permanent ban
Arrhythmias	If symptomatic while driving. Driving may continue once symptoms are controlled	Yes	
Occasional ventricular premature beats	No restrictions	No	
Frequent or polymorphic premature beats	Stop driving, pending CVS investigation	Yes	Check with DVLC
Ventricular tachycardia	Stop driving, pending CVS investigation Driving may continue once symptoms are controlled with annual review	Yes	
Implanted defibrillator	Avoid driving forever	Yes	
CNS disorders	Where definite diagnosis of progressive disability; refer to DVLC for specific advice with consent of patient	Yes	Check with DVLC
Complete heart block	Driving forbidden until 1 month after pacing	Yes	Forbidden
Conduction abnormalities	If symptomatic avoid driving pending CVS investigation Can drive when symptoms are controlled	Yes	Check with DVLC

Congenital heart anomalies	No restrictions unless arrhythmia, angina or syncope Post-surgery, 1 month	No No	Check with DVLC
Congenital heart block (usually bradycardia)	3 year licence after CVS investigation, including stress test and 24-hour ECG, repeated annually	Yes	Usually forbidden
Diabetes	Can hold licence for 1, 2 or 3 years depending on complications and diabetic type IDDM patients need to demonstrate: • Understanding of disease • Reasonable control • No frequent or unexplained hypoglycaemic attacks *Always carry sugar in car*	Yes	Need to notify DVLC if becomes IDDM, with individual review Established IDDM will not be granted new vocational licences
Drugs (if any side effects which impair consciousness or motor response)	Avoid driving while taking drug Warn patient that alcohol potentiates side effects of many drugs	No	
Epilepsy	Can hold (renewable) licence for up to 3 years *if:* • Free of fits for 2 years • Fits only while asleep for 3 years • Avoid for 6 months during treatment changes	Yes Yes Yes	Allowed if fit free since 5 years of age *or* Fit free for 10 years and off medication *and* seeing neurologist annually to confirm fit-free status

continued on p. 222

Fitness to drive (*continued*)

Condition	Normal licence	Notification of DVLC	Vocational licence
Single fit	• Cannot drive until investigated • Possible 1-year ban	Yes	See previous comment for driving post-fit
Hypertension (uncomplicated)	No restriction	No	
Impaired locomotor system	Avoid driving. If permanent disability, refer to DVLC	Yes	Refer to DVLC
MI	Avoid driving for 1 month	No	Many restrictions; refer to DVLC
Pacemakers	Can hold licence for up to 3 years 1 month post-implantation *if*: • Followed up annually • Asymptomatic	Yes	Refer to DVLC
PVD	No restriction		
Syncope, TIA, LOC	Avoid driving until problem solved; 3 month ban	Yes	Permanent ban
Valvular heart disease	No restrictions if no arrhythmia, angina or syncope	No	Check with DVLC

From Raffel A. (ed.) (1985) *Medical Aspects of Fitness to Drive: a Guide for Medical Practitioners*. Medical Commission on Accident Prevention, London.

Appendix B: Diagrams for explaining procedures to patients

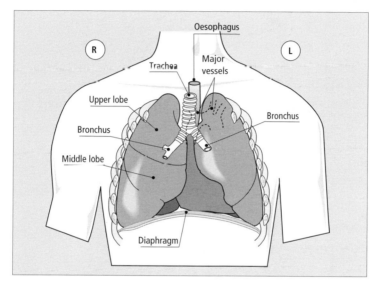

Fig. A1 The thorax. For example:
- Bronchoscopy.
- Chest surgery.

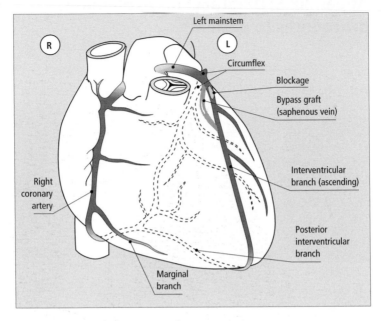

Fig. A2 Coronary arteries. For example:
• CABG.

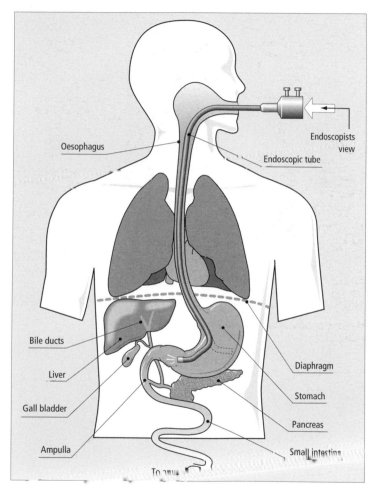

Fig. A3 Upper gastrointestinal tract. For example:
- Upper endoscopy (± ERCP).
- Liver biopsy.
- Cholecystectomy/biliary surgery.
- Pancreatitis.
- Gall stones.

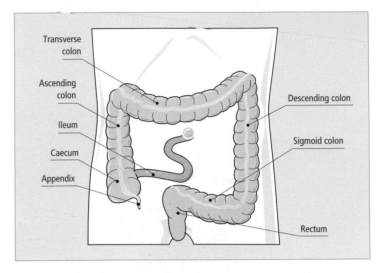

Fig. A4 Large intestine. For example:
- Colonoscopy.
- Large bowel surgery.
- Diverticular disease.
- Colonic carcinoma.

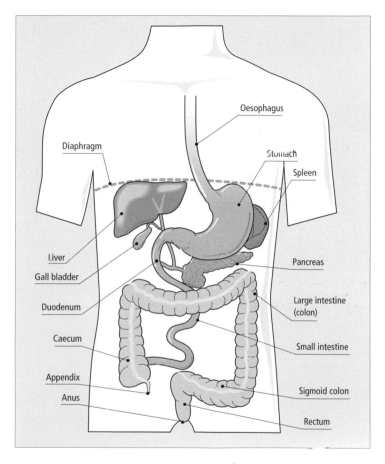

Fig. A5 Digestive organs — schematic (small intestine is much longer than in diagram, for example.
- Major abdominal surgery.
- Intestinal disorders.

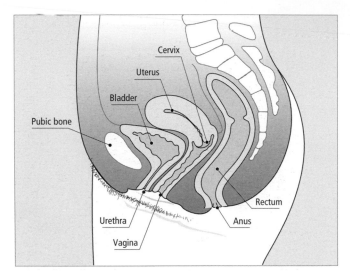

Fig. A6 Female pelvis. For example:
• Catheterization.
• Gynaecological disorders.

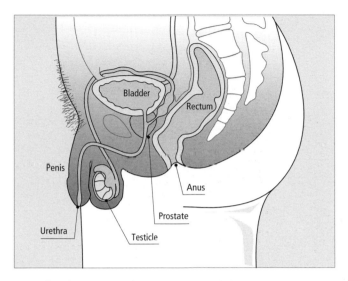

Fig. A7 Male pelvis. For example:
- Catheterization.
- Prostatectomy.

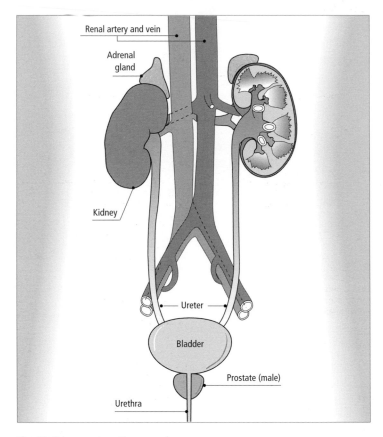

Fig. A8 Urinary system. For example:
- Renal biopsy.
- Renal stones.
- Bladder disorders.

Index

Page numbers in *italics* indicate figures; those in **bold** indicate tables.

abdominal pain 22, 39–40, 51, 59
  acute 114
  pain relief 40, **138**
  pregnant women 22
abdominal plain films 180–1
abdominal surgery 191, *227*
ABGs *see* arterial blood gases (ABGs)
abstracts 25
accident and emergency 16–22
  admitting patients 16–17
  medical conditions 17
  pain relief 21
  patient information organization 17
  surgical conditions 21–2
accident forms 8, 11–12
accommodation 198
ACE inhibitors 57, 71, 79
acetylcysteine (Parvolex) 19, *20*
acid–base disorders 144
acidosis 19, 76, 78, 143, 144
acne 81, 115
actinic keratoses 81
acupuncture 138
acute red eyes 56
acyclovir 116
Addisonian crisis 116, 195
Addison's disease 72, 79, 84, 116
Additional Voluntary Contributions (AVCs)
      209
addresses 215
adenomas 128
adenosine 44
ADH (antidiuretic hormone) 85
  inappropriate 110
  A&E patients 16–17
  GP communication 30
adrenal insufficiency 72
adrenal suppression 116
adrenaline 72, 75, 87, 106, 107, 128–9
  in local anaesthesia 165
Advanced Life Support (ALS) 35
  protocol *36*
aggression, and dying patients 91

agranulocytosis 82
AIDS *see* HIV/AIDS
albumin deficit 45, 46
alcohol abuse 62
alcohol consumption 129
  limits 109
alcohol withdrawal 49, 58, 61, 109–10, 111
alcoholism 50, 109–10, 128
alkalosis 79, 80, 81, 83, 143
allergies 113, 185
allopurinol 58
ALS (Advanced Life Support) 35
alternative careers 198–9
aluminium-based drugs 50
amaurosis fugax 57
amiloride 79
aminoglycosides 60, 154
aminophylline poisoning 19
amiodarone 43, **108**
amitriptyline 73–4
amoxicillin 105
amphetamines, overdose 61
amphotericin B 79
ampicillin 105
amputation 160, 191
anaemia 40–1, 49, 57
  blood transfusions 40–1, 85, 86
  investigations 130
  sickle cell 114–15
anaesthetics 57, 110, 123, 124, 170, 190
  creams 150
  surgical patients 191–2
  and hypotension 161
analgesia 40, 70, 73, 78, 114
  opiate 72, 107
  postoperative 196
  and terminal care 93
analgesics 49, 133–9
anaphylaxis 71, 72, 74, 75, 82, 87
  and anticoagulation 106
  drug-induced 107
  and intravenous drug administration
      103

angina 19, 47, 48, 105, 161
angioplasty 121, 122
anorexia 21
antacids 40, 46, 50, 51
anti-arrhythmics 45
antibiotics 51, 58, 59, 67, 72, 78
  and central lines 154
  intravenous administration 103
  perioperative prescribing 186, 191
  protocols 105
  and sickle cell anaemia 114
  side effects 60, 105
anticholinergics 50
  poisoning 19
anticoagulant therapy 64
anticoagulants 121
anticoagulation 64, 67, 68
  perioperative prescribing 186–9
  protocol 105–6
antidepressants 135
  see also tricyclic antidepressants
antidiuretic hormone (ADH), secreting
    tumour 85
anti-emetics 76, 83
antihistamines 74
antihypertensives 71
anti-inflammatory steroids 115
antipyretics 59–60
anuria 87–8
anxiety 51, 73, 135
aortic aneurysm 47
  repair 191
aortic dissection 47
aortic stenosis 161
aortic valve disease 127
appendicitis 114
Apple Macintosh (computers) 23
application forms 205
arrhythmias 57, 58, 75, 80, 83, 88
  bradyarrhythmias 43
  hypotension 71
  management 42–5
  tachyarrhythmias 44–5
  uncontrolled 161
arterial blood gases (ABGs) 45, 66, 77–8, 80,
    132
  arterial puncture procedure 140–5
  arterial puncture sites 141
  interpretation 142–5
  pH 143–4
  P_{O_2} 142–3
  serum electrolytes 144

type 1 respiratory failure (pink puffers)
    144–5
type 2 respiratory failure (blue bloaters)
    145
arteriography 183
ascites, investigations 129–30
aspiration pneumonia 105
aspirin 101, 133
  poisoning 19
asthma 82, 83, 84, 176
atrial fibrillation 28, 42, 43, 44, 52, 53
atrial flutter 44, 53
atrial tachycardia 44, 53
atrioventricular (AV) heart block 42, 43, 45
atrioventricular (AV) nodal rhythm 53
atropine 43, 140, 173
attention seeking, and terminal care 91
AVCs (Additional Voluntary Contributions)
    209

bacterial infections 82, 115
bad news 90–1
  information for patients' families 32, 33
bank nurses 31
banking 211
barium 123, 183
  enemas 124, 178, 182
barium meal 182
barium swallows 129, 182
Barthel Activities Index 5, 215–16
basal cell carcinomas 81, 82
baseline tests 17, 21
basic emergency routine 88–9
BBB (bundle branch block) 45
bed allocation 17
bedpans 50
benzodiazepines 50, 69, 73–4
  addiction 73
bereavement officers 96
beta-blockers 43, 70, 72, 161
betadine 162, 164, 166
beta-lactams 60
bibliographic databases 24, 26
bibliography 2–3
bicarbonate 79, 132
biliary cirrhosis 129
biliary peritonitis 125
biliary surgery 191, *225*
bilirubin 61
biochemical formulae 219
biochemistry, results 218–19
biochemistry samples 18

biochemistry tubes 107
bisacodyl 51
bladder catheterization 145–6
    men 145–6
    women 146
bladder disorders *230*
bleeps (pagers) 6, 31, 38, 199
blood cultures 59, 60, 146–7
blood forms 4, 8, 12–13
blood glucose tests 48
blood groups 86
blood letting 147–8
blood requests 12–13
blood samples
    haemophiliacs 112
    HIV/AIDS patients 112–13
blood stains 3, 200
blood transfusions 85–6
    anaemia 40–1
    and fever 58, 59
    upper gastrointestinal bleeds 64, 65
blue bloaters 145
BMJ *see British Medical Journal* (BMJ)
body fluids, electrolytes **63**
bolus injection 136
bone marrow biopsies 41, 190
bone pain relief **138**
bony metastases 46, 184
books 2–3
bowel infarction 40
bowel resection 190
brachial artery puncture 141
bradyarrhythmias 43
bradycardia 43, 71, 72, 166
brain abscess 69
British Medical Association (BMA) 28, 37,
        199, 205, 212
    Internet access 200, 201
    junior doctor representatives 213
    newspaper cuttings database 27
British Medical Journal (BMJ) 25, 199
    Classifieds 202, 206
    (*Minor*) *Economee 2*)
    Evidence-Based Medicine 26
British National Formulary (BNF) 18, 93,
        106, 138, 204
    and drug prescribing 99, 101, 105, 189
bronchopneumonia 131–2
bronchoscopy *223*
bulk-forming agents 51
bullous impetigo 81
bullying 212

bundle branch block (BBB) 45, 55
bupivacaine 163, 165
burial 95
Buscopan **138**

café-au-lait spots 81
CAGE questionnaire 109
calcitonin 46
calcium 45–7
calcium channel blockers 43, 50
calcium gluconate 47, 79
calcium phosphate 46
Calcium Resonium (polystyrene sulphonate
        resin) 79
calcium-based drugs 50
Candida 113, 115, 116
candidiasis 81, 105, 191
Canesten 116
cannulae 110, 126, 150–1, 153–5, 171–3,
        192
    sizes **149**
cannulation
    procedures 148–51
    right internal jugular vein 151, 153
    subclavian vein 151, 153
carbamazepine 19, **108, 138**
carbenicillin 79
carbohydrate intolerance 66
carbon dioxide, levels 77–8
carcinomas 81, 82, 85
    colonic *226*
cardiac arrests 35–7, 64
    protocol *36*
cardiac catheterization 121–2
    complications 122
cardiac enzymes 127
cardiac tamponade 173
cardiological investigations 127–8
cardiomyopathy 71, 161
cardiopulmonary resuscitation (CPR)
        35–7
    complications 11, 1*, 121–3
    complications 123
    procedures 158–9
careers
    alternative 198–9
    consultants 205, 206
    see also jobs
carotid sinus massage 45
carpopedal spasm 47
cars 199
CASES 185

CASH (chest, abdomen, systemic, head) 74, **75**
catecholamines 128–9, 156
catheterization *228–9*
catheters 46, 64, 68, 88, 89, 145–6
  changing 22
  heart 121
  peritoneal 170
CCF (congestive cardiac failure) 84
CD-ROMs 23, 27
cefuroxime 105, 107
cell lysis 79
cellulitis 105
central lines 151–7
  CVP measurement 155–7
  insertion 151–4
  jugular approach 151–2
  temporary 154–5
  tunneled lines 154–5
  useage 155
central pontine myelinolysis 85
central retinal vein/artery occlusion 57
central venous pressure (CVP), measurement 155–7
cephalosporins 105
cerebellar disease 57
cerebrovascular accident (CVA) 61
  head CT 183
charge nurses 31
chemotherapy 76, 77, 82, 155
cherry angiomas 82
chest, abdomen, systemic, head (CASH) 74, **75**
chest drains 157–8
  insertion 157–8
  removal 158
chest infection 105
chest pain 44, 47–8, 59, 71, 127
  pleuritic **138**, 162
chest surgery *223*
chest X-rays 45, 48, 83, 115, 154, 173
  and pacemakers 97
  preoperative 180, 192
chicken pox 81
children 110
  consent 110, 190, 196
  dental charting 196
  drug prescribing 99
  oro-facio-maxillary surgery 196–7
  terminal care 92
chloral hydrate 73
chlorpheniramine (chlorphenamine) 72, 74, 75, 86, 87

chlorpromazine 49, 50
chlorpropamide 84
cholecalciferol 47
cholecystectomy *225*
cholecystitis 47
cholesterol 127, 128
Christian Scientists 113–14
chronic obstructive airways disease (COAD) 77–8, 82, 83, 132, 176
Chvostek's sign 47
cimetidine 51
ciprofloxacin 105
cirrhosis 64, 84, 171
CL (Cochrane Library) 27, 28
clerking 17
  day surgery 196
  medical patients 117
  surgical patients 185–6, 197
clinical stalemate 118–21
clomethiazole 49, 50, 62, 109–10
Clostridium difficile 51, 52, 105, 129
clothes 199–200
clotrimazole 116
clotting factors 86
cluster headaches 69
COAD (chronic obstructive airways disease) 77–8, 82, 83, 132, 176
Cochrane Library (CL) 27, 28
co-codamol 139
co-danthrusate 51
codeine 67, 138
  side effects 135
codeine phosphate 139
co-dydramol **138**
colchicine 51
cold sores 116
colitis 124
colleagues, contacting 200
colloid fluid replacement 64, 75
colonic carcinomas *226*
colonic surgery 191
colonic tumours 41
colonoscopy 124, *226*
colostomy 190, 191
coma, unexplained 130–1
common calls 38–89
Communicable Disease Surveillance Centre 217
communication 28–33, 37
  bad news 32, 33, 90–1
  consultants 29–30
  dying patients 90–3
  GPs 30

communication (*continued*)
  nurses 30–2, 94
  patients 32, 38
  patients' families 32–3, 37, 91, 95
  senior registrars 29–30
  terminal care 90–3
  see also information-giving
communications software 24–5, 26
compassionate leave 202
computerized tomography (CT) 180, **181**,
    183
computers 23–6
  hardware 23–4
  Internet 23, 25–6
  online database access 25
  software 23, 24–5, 26
concussion 49
conditions of service 200–4
condylomata acuminata 81
confidentiality 33–4
conflict management 29
confusion 47, 48–50, 73
congestive cardiac failure (CCF) 84
conjunctivitis 56
consent 122–3
  children 110, 190, 196
  surgical patients 189–91, 196
consent forms 8
constipation 50–1, 79, 191
consultants 4
  career prospects 205, 206
  communication 29–30
continuing medical education 23
contracts 199, 200–4
  compassionate leave 202
  holiday entitlement 202
  maternity/paternity leave 202
  notice 202
  occupational health requirements 203–4
  overtime 201–2
  pay 199, 201–2
  rotas 200–1
  sick leave 203
  study leave 203
contrast studies 181–2
controlled drugs 100–2
coping problems 212–13
co-proxamol 67, 138–9
corneal ulceration 56
coronary arteries *224*
coronary artery spasm (variant angina) 55
coroners 95, 96–7
corticosteroids 66

cortisol 128
cortisone 107
costochondritis 48
counselling services 212
COX-2 (cyclo-oxygenase type-2) inhibitors
    135
crash calls 35–7
creatinine 64, 70, 88, 131
cremation 94, 95
cremation fees 97–8, 204
  tax 97
cremation forms 94, 97–8
Crown Indemnity 208
CRUSE 93
Cryptococcus 130
Cryptosporidium 52, 60
CT (computerized tomography) 180, **181**,
    183
curriculum vitae (CV) 205–6
Cushing's disease/syndrome 128
Cushing's reflex 71
CV (curriculum vitae) 205–6
CVA (cerebrovascular accident) 61
CVP (central venous pressure) 155–7
cyanosis 88
cyclizine lactate 77
cyclo-oxygenase type-2 (COX-2) inhibitors
    135
cytotoxic agents 51, 84, 101

daily patient notes 11
danthron docusate 51
databases 24, 25, 27
day surgery 196
DC cardioversion *see* cardioversion
death 94–8
  clinical confirmation 94
  cremation forms 97–8
  informing relatives 95
  referral to coroner/procurator fiscal 96–7
  registration 96–7
  relatives 95
  what to do 94
death certificates 94, 95–6, 97
  occupation-related deaths 96
  war-related deaths 96
deep vein thrombosis (DVT) 105
defibrillators 35
dehydration 16, 46, 50, 72, 76
  and alcoholism 109
dementia 49, 111
dental charting 196
Department of Health 206

depression 21, 73, 110–11, 113, 128, 135
  in doctors 203, 212
dermatitis
  atopic 82
  contact 82
dermatitis herpetiformis 81
desks 6
desk-top publishing 25
dexamethasone 107, 128
dextropropoxyphene 139
dextrose 47, 62–3, 66, 86, 101, 111
  infusion 80
diabetes mellitus 56, 58, 59, 162
  glucose, potassium, insulin regime **194**
  investigations 128
  and steroids 115
  surgical patients 193–5
  surgical protocols **194**
diabetic coma 101
diabetic ketoacidosis (DKA) 66, 79
diabetic neuropathy **138**
diamorphine 83, 136, 137, **138**
diarrhoea 51–2, 59, 79, 105, 113, 191
  explosive 124
  investigations 129
diazepam 49, 50, 61, 168
DIC (disseminated intravascular coagulation)
    130
diclofenac 135, **138**
diclofenac sodium (Voltarol) 21
diflunisal 135
digestive organs *227*
digoxin 43, 44, 51, 69, 76, 80
  administration protocol 106–7
  side effects 106
  therapeutic drug levels **108**
  toxicity 45, 55, 107, 122
dihydrocodeine 135
diphenhydramine 77
discharge 4, 6
  day surgery 196
  GP communication 30
  information for patients' families 32–3
discharge letters 30
discharge summaries 4, 6, 8, 13–14
dissecting aneurysm 48
disseminated intravascular coagulation (DIC)
    130
diuretics 79, 107
diverticular disease 52, *226*
diverticulitis 124
DKA (diabetic ketoacidosis) 66, 79

'do not resuscitate' orders 37
Doctors and Dentists' Review Body 201
doctors' mess 198, 204, 213
docusate sodium 51
domperidone 77
dopamine 102
dopamine agonists 76
doxapram 78
dress 3
Dressler's syndrome 47
driving, fitness 220–2
droperidol 77
drug administration 101–5
  infusions 99, 102–3
  intravenous drugs 103–5
drug charts 4, 8, 16, 39, 52, 99–100
  verbal requests 101
drug infusions 99, 102–3
drug overdose *see* overdose
drug prescribing 99–101
  abbreviations **100**
  children 99
  controlled drugs 100–2
  elderly patients 99
  infusions 99, 102
  terminal care 93, 99
  verbal requests 101
  written prescriptions 100
drug representatives 204
Drug and Therapeutics Bulletin 204
drug withdrawal 61, 111
drug-induced headaches 69
drugs 49, 99–108
  blood levels 107
  inhaled 133
  oral 133–6
  therapeutic levels 107, **108**
dry skin 74
DVT (deep vein thrombosis) 105
dying *see* death
dying patients
  aggression 91
  communication 90–3
  questions to ask 92
dyshidrosis 81
dysmenorrhoea 67
dyspepsia 115
dysphagia 115
dyspnoea 161

E-45 74
echocardiography 127, 128

ectopic pregnancy 67
eczema, dyshidrotic 82
elderly patients 111
  confusion 48
  drug prescribing 99
  falls 57–8
  intravenous fluids 63
electrocardiogram (ECG) 52–6
  abnormalities 55–6
  arrhythmias 42–4
  chest pain 47–8
  lead placement 159, *160*
  parameters 53
  procedures 159–60
electrolyte imbalance 62, 76, 111
  and alcoholism 109
  crash calls 35
  elderly patients 111
electrolytes
  body fluids **63**
  serum 144
email 200
Emla anaesthetic cream 150
empyema 157, 173
  chest drains insertion 158
encephalitis 69
endocarditis 118, 146
  investigations 128
  subacute bacterial 60
endocrinological investigations 128–9
endocrinopathies 46
endometriosis 67
endoscopy 123–4, 129, *225*
enemas 51, 178, 182
Entonox 133, **136**
epidermoid cysts 81
epilepsy 61, 62
equipment 3–4, 16, 39
erythema multiforme bullosum 81
erythemas 81–2
erythromycin 105
euphoria 115
  and hypoxia 83, 111
euthanasia 206
evidence-based medicine 26, 27–8
examinations, medical patients 118,
  120
exercise stress test 161
expenses 209
exsanguinating bleed 35
eye complaints 56–7
  acute red eyes 56

floaters 57
sudden loss of vision 57
eye surgery 4

face-masks 72, 77
facial bruising 78
faecal impaction 51
faecal retention 49
falls 49, 57–8
fatigue
  doctors 1, 203, 213
  postoperative 190
female pelvis *228*
femoral artery puncture 141, *143*
fentanyl 186
ferrous sulphate 50
fetuses 114
FEV (forced expiratory volume) **174**, 175
fever 58–60, 105, 113
  postoperative causes **59**
fibroids 67
financial advice 199
firm timetables 10
fitness to drive 220–2
fits 60–2
flexible training 213
floaters 57
flucloxacillin 60, 78, 105
fluconazole 116
fluid charts 4, 8, 16, 39, **62**, 63
fluid overload 111
  central venous pressure (CVP) 156
folate 114
folliculitis 81
forced expiratory volume (FEV) **174**, 175
forced vital capacity (FVC) 175
forms 8
  accident and emergency 16
  information management 8–10
formulae, biochemical 219
fractures 12, 111
frusemide vi
furosemide (frusemide) 46, 83, 86
furunculosis cellulitis 82
FVC (forced vital capacity) 175

G&S (group and save) 186
gall stones *225*
gastric lavage 18, 19
gastritis 39, 40, 47, 76
gastroenteritis 76
gastroenterological investigations 129–30

Gastrografin 183
gastrointestinal bleeds
  investigations 129
  lower GI tract 65
  upper GI tract 63–5
General Medical Council (GMC) 200
  registration 202
genito-urinary surgery 191
gentamicin 105, **108**
geography of hospital 4
GKI (glucose, potassium, insulin) regime
     193, **194**
Glasgow Coma Scale 57, 131, 216
glaucoma 4
  acute 56, 57, 69
glucagon 66, 75
glucocorticoids, side effects 115
glucose 79, 193
  levels 195
glucose abnormalities 65–6
glucose, potassium, insulin (GKI) regime
     193, **194**
glucose samples 18, 19
glucose tolerance test 161–2
glycerine suppositories 51
glyceryl trinitrate (GTN) 48
  continuous infusions 102
GMC (General Medical Council) 200, 202
GP liaison 30
  accident and emergency admissions 16–17
  death 94
  discharge summary 13
granisetron 77
granuloma annulare 82
granulomatous diseases 46
grief 111
Groschong lines 155
group and save (G&S) 186
GTN (glyceryl trinitrate) 48, 102
gynaecological disorders 66–7, *228*

Haemaccel 64, 72, 75
haematemesis 64, 65
haematological investigations 130
haematology, results 218
haematuria 67–8, 70, 126, 127
haemoglobinopathies 41
haemolysis 68, 148
haemophiliacs 111–12
haemoptysis 65
haemorrhage 124, 126, 168, 171
haemorrhoidectomy 191

hacmorrhoids 50
haemothorax 157
  chest drain insertion 158
haloperidol 49, 50, 84
hand backs 14
handovers 14
hardware 23–4
HASH CREDIT 185
head injury
  head CT **181**, 183
  skull X-ray 180, **181**
headaches 68–70
  pain relief **138**
  post-lumbar puncture 168
Health Trends 206
heart block 45, 52, 55, 72
heart failure 41, 42–3, 44, 70, 105
  investigations 127
heartburn 116
heparin 102, 105–6, 152, 186, 189
  arterial blood samples 141
heparinization 121
hepatic coma 110
hepatic failure 125
hepatitis B 129, 130, 140
  haemophiliacs 111–12
  immunization status 204
  needlestick injuries 212
hepatitis C 129, 130
  haemophiliacs 111–12
  needlestick injuries 212
Hepsal 103, 154
herpes simplex 81
herpes zoster 115
herpetic keratitis 56
Hickman lines 155
history sheets 8, 16, 17, 185–6
history taking 5
  medical background 117
  medical patients 117–21
  surgical patients 185–6
  systematic (functional) enquiry 118
HIV testing 85, 113
  following needlestick injuries 211–12
HIV/AIDS 52
  haemophiliacs 112
  needlestick injuries 211–12
  patient care 112–13
  taking blood 112–13
Hodgkin's lymphoma 74
holiday entitlement 202
hospices 93

hospital layout 4
5-HT₃ antagonists 77
hydrocortisone 46, 107, 115, 195
    and anaphylaxis 72, 75
    and transfusions 86, 87
hyoscine butylbromide 138
hypercalcaemia 45–6, 50
hypercarbia 77, 78
hyperglycaemia 57, 66
hyperkalaemia 63, 65, 79, 111
hyperparathyroidism 46
hypertension 70–1, 115
    investigations 127–8
    malignant 70
hypertensive encephalopathy 69
hyperthyroidism 58
hyperventilation 83
    spurious hypocalcaemia 46
hypoalbuminaemia 45
hypocalcaemia 46–7
hypoglycaemia 16, 18, 65–6, 75, 88
    and alcoholism 109
    and confusion 49
    and diabetes 193
    and falls 57
    and fits 61
hypokalaemia 50, 65–6, 79–81, 107, 115
hypomagnesaemia 80
hyponatraemia 63, 84–5
hypotension 44, 71–2, 75, 82, 87, 88
    and alcoholism 109
    and falls 57, 58
    and fits 61
    surgical patients 195
hypothermia 43, 88, 111
hypothyroidism 43, 46, 50, 51, 84
    investigations 129
hypoventilation 77
hypovolaemia 44, 88, 114, 151
    central venous pressure (CVP) 156
    hypotension 71, 72
    upper gastrointestinal (GI) bleed 113, 114, 116
hypoxia 49, 61, 77, 78, 83, 88
    and depression 111
    elderly patients 48, 111
    and euphoria 83, 111

IBD (inflammatory bowel disease) 51, 52
IBS (irritable bowel syndrome) 50
ibuprofen 58, 67, 70, 78, 135
IDDM (insulin-dependent diabetes mellitus) 194

IHD see ischaemic heart disease (IHD)
ileostomy 190, 191
ileus 50
illness, in doctors 203
iMac (computer) 23
immunization status 204
immunocompromised host
    diarrhoea 51, 52
    fever 60
income protection 208
individual savings accounts (ISAs) 210–11
infection
    confusion 49
    postoperative 191
infestations 74
inflammatory bowel disease (IBD) 51, 52, 58
information-giving
    breaking bad news 32, 33
    confidentiality 33–4
    day surgery 196
    diagrams 190, 223–30
    patients' families 32–3
    preparation for procedures 190
    surgical patients 190–1, 196
infusion pumps 93, 102
inhaled drugs 133
initiative 2
injections
    intramuscular 162, 163
    joint 157, 164–5
    subcutaneous 162
Inland Revenue 209–10
insect bites 82
insomnia 21, 72–4
insulin 65–6, 79
    infusion 194–5
    sliding scale 195
insulin therapy, diabetic surgical patients 193–5
insulin-dependent diabetes mellitus (IDDM) 194
insurance
    car 199
    room contents 204–5
intensive therapy unit (ITU) 186
intercostal blocks 162–3, 165
internal jugular vein cannulation 151, 153
Internet 23, 25–6, 200, 201
interpreters 29, 91
interstitial renal disease 84
interviews 206
intestinal disorders 227

intestinal fistulae 79
intestinal obstruction 39, 50, 51, 76
intracranial pressure elevation 43, 69, 76
intramuscular injections 162, *163*
intraperitoneal bleeding 41
intravenous drug administration 103–5
   liquid drugs 103
   powdered drugs 103–5
intravenous fluids 62–3
   prescription 62–3
intravenous urography 181–2
investigations
   cardiology 127–8
   endocrinology 128–9
   gastroenterology 129–30
   haematology 130
   neurology 130–1
   radiology 178
   renal medicine 131
   respiratory medicine 131–2
   rheumatology 132
iritis, acute 56
irritable bowel syndrome (IBS) 50
ISAs (individual savings accounts) 210–11
ischaemic heart disease (IHD) 45, 47, 48,
   159
   investigations 127
isoprenaline 43
itching 74

JAMA (*Journal of the American Medical
   Association*) 25, 28
jargon, avoidance 32
jaundice 43, 74, 125
   surgical patients 191, 193
Jehovah's witnesses 113–14
job interviews 206
jobs 205–7
   consultant career prospects 205, 206
   interviews 206
   locums 206–7
   referees 205
   see also careers
joint aspiration 163–4
joint injections 157, 164–5
Journal of the American Medical Association
   (JAMA) 25, 28
journals 25, 26–7
junior doctors
   hospital committees 198, 213
   representation 213

Junior Doctors' Committee 200
Junior Doctors' New Deal 199, 200, 213
   hours **201**

keratisis, acute 56
ketoacidosis 193
ketoconazole 113
ketones 66
keyboards (computers) 24

lactic acid 148
lactulose 51
laparoscopic surgery 189, 190
laparotomy 130
lap-top computers 24
large bowel surgery *226*
large intestine *226*
laryngospasm 47
laundry 199–200
laxatives 50, 51, 79, 107, 108, 182
LBBB (left bundle branch block) 55, 161
leave 202–3
lecturer practitioners 31
left bundle branch block (LBBB) 55, 161
left ventricular failure (LVF) 73, 82, 83
left ventricular hypertrophy (LVH) 55
legal aspects
   confidentiality 33–4
   day surgery case discharge 196
lentigines 81
leukaemia 82
leukoerythroblastic anaemia 41
lichen planus 82
lidocaine 141, 163, 165, 166, 171
line insertion 148–51
lipomas 81
lists 8–10
literature, keeping up to date 26–7
lithium **108**
liver biopsy 125, *225*
liver failure 49
   investigations 130
living wills 37
local anaesthesia 126, 165
locums 14, 206–7
long-term illness income protection 208
lorazepam 50, 109
lower gastrointestinal tract
   bleeds 65
   investigations 129
lumbar puncture 166–8

lumen, blocked 154
lupus erythematosus 82
LVF (left ventricular failure) 73, 82, 83
LVH (left ventricular hypertrophy) 55
lymph node drainage 78

MacMillan Nurses 93–4
magnesium citrate 124
magnesium deficiency 47
magnesium sulphate 51
magnetic resonance imaging (MRI) 131, 184
malaise 69
male pelvis 229
malignant disease 46, 84
malignant hypertension 70
malnutrition, elderly patients 111
Mantoux test 132, 168–9
Marcain 165
Marie Curie Cancer Care 94
marking surgical patients 192
mastectomy 191
maternity leave 202
meals 207
measles 115
Med 3 form 15
medical colleagues, contacting 200
medical defence 34, 37, 207–8
medical emergencies 17
medical ethics 37
medical patients
  clerking 117
  examination 118
  history taking 117–21
  medical background 117
  preparation for procedures 121–7
  specialist referrals/investigations 127–32
Medicalert bracelets 126
MEDLINE 25, 27, 28
mefenamic acid 67
melaena 64, 65
melanomas 81, 82

alcohol limits 109
bladder catheterization 145–6
meningism 59, 69
  investigations 130
meningitis 61, 69, 70, 130, 166
menorrhagia 41
menstrual bleeding 67
Mental Health Act 97, 216–17
  self-discharge prevention 15

mental illness
  in doctors 203
  and steroids 115
meprobamate 138
metabolic disorders 49, 50, 61, 76, 79
metadrenalines 129
metal implants, check before MRI 184
methicillin resistant Staphylococcus aureus
  (MRSA) 204
methylcellulose 79
methylprednisolone 165
metoclopramide 77, 83
metronidazole 60, 105, 107
MI see myocardial infarction (MI)
mice (computers) 24
miconazole 113, 116
Microsoft Word 24
migraine 69, 70, 76
mineralocorticoids
  deficiency 79
  excess 79
  side effects 115
mini-mental test 49, 57, 217
minors, consent 190, 196
mithramycin 46
mitral/aortic stenosis 57
modems 23, 25, 26
moisturizers 74
molluscum contagiosum 81
money management 208–11
  income protection 208
  payslip deductions 208
  pensions 209
  tax 209–11
monitors (computers) 24
mood change 111
moribund patients 74–6
morphine 135, 138, 186, 193
  continuous infusions 102, 137
motor dysfunction 57
MRI (magnetic resonance imaging) 131, 184
MRSA (methicillin resistant Staphylococcus
  aureus) 204
multiple sclerosis 57
muscle wasting 115
myalgia 69
mycobacteria 52
Mycobacterium tuberculosis 168
mycosis fungoides 82
myelodysplasia 86
myeloma 46, 130

myocardial infarction (MI) 13, 43, 44, 75,
83
acute 47
chest pain 47
crash calls 35
elderly patients 111
electrocardiogram 52, 55–6
hypotension 71
investigations 127
pain relief **138**
myocarditis 47, 55, 71
myoglobinuria 68

naevi 81
naloxone 75, 138
naproxen 133, 135, **138**
narcosis 77, 78
nasal specs 77
nasogastric tubes (NGTs) 169, 190–1
National Insurance 208
nausea 52, 76–7
necrobiosis lipoidicum 81
needlestick injuries 30, 211–12
neoplasm 51
nephritis 127
nephrotic syndrome 84, 85
investigations 131
nerve blockades 138
netilmicin 105
neuralgia 135
neurological investigations 130–1
next of kin, notification 94, 95, 96
NGTs (nasogastric tubes) 169, 190–1
nicotine 44, 109
NIDDM (non-insulin dependent diabetes
mellitus) 66, 193–4
nifedipine 70
night rounds 5–6
night sedation 107
nitrates 44, 69, 71
nodal (junctional) supraventricular
tachycardia 44
nodules 81, 82
non-insulin dependent diabetes mellitus
(NIDDM) 66, 193–4
non-steroidal anti-inflammatory drugs
(NSAIDs) 67, 70, 76, 133–6
pros/cons **136**
noradrenaline 128–9
'not for resus' 37
notice 202
notifiable diseases 217–18

NSAIDs (non-steroidal anti-inflammatory
drugs) 67, 70, 76, 133–6
nurse managers 31
nurses 1
communication 30–2, 94
drug administration 101, 102–3
grades 31
liability 11, 57
nasogastric tube insertion 169
shifts 31–2
and terminal care 90, 91
verbal drug requests 101
nystatin 113, 116

obesity 128
obstructive lung disease, investigations 132
occult bleeding 41
occult pain 111
occupational health requirements 203–4
oesophageal spasm 47, 48
oesophageal varices 64
oesophagitis 47, 76
oliguria 87–8
ondansetron 77
on-line banking 211
operations, preoperative checklist **188–9**, 192
ophthalmic examination 4, 56
ophthalmoscopes 3–4
opiate analgesia 72, 107
opiates 49, 50, 51
antidote 138
bolus injection 136
infusions 137
nausea/vomiting 76
oral 136
overdose 19, 75
pain relief in addicts 21
pros/cons **137**
and terminal care 93
optic neuritis 57
oral contraceptives 67, 105, 189
oral drugs 133–6
organization of paperwork 4, 8–10, 11–15, 17
orientation day 1
oro-facio-maxillary surgery 196–7
orthopnoea 73
osteoporosis 115
overdose 17–21, 35
fits 61
history taking 21
patient assessment 18–19
treatment refusal 20

overdose (*continued*)
  washouts 18, 19
overhead presentation software 24
overtime 201–2
oxazepam 73
oxygen therapy 77–8

P waves 52, 53–4, 55, 158
pacemakers
  checks
    before cremation 94, 97
    before MRI 184
  insertion 125–6
paediatric blood bottles 110
pain 51, 126, 133–9
  acute 135
  chronic 135
  constipation 50
  emotional component *134*, 135
  period 67
  phantom limb **138**
  physical component *134*, 134–5
  and sleep 73
  stimulus-independent 134–5
  see also abdominal pain; chest pain
pain relief 133–9
  accident and emergency 21
  categorization 138–9
  common clinical conditions **138**
  hypertension 70
  mild pain **137**
  moderate pain **137**
  opiate addicts 21
  severe pain **137**
  terminal care 91, 93
palm-held computers 24
pancreatitis 46, 47, *225*
papaveretum 136, **138**
papaverine 136
paperwork organization 4, 8–10, 11–15, 17
papilloedema 166
p⟨ ⟩ l⟨⟩ 01⟨ 0⟩
paracentesis (peritoneal tap) 169–71
paracetamol 70, 87, 101, 108, 125, 139
  as antipyretic 59–60
  applications **138**
  poisoning 18, 19
  pros/cons **136**
paraesthesia 47
paraneoplastic syndrome 46
paranoid psychosis 115
paraphimosis 146

paraprotein investigation 130
Parkinson's disease 57, 160
paroxysmal nocturnal dyspnoea (PND) 73
part-time work 213
Parvolex (acetylcysteine) 19, *20*
paternity leave 202
patient notes 5, 11, 12–13, 92
patients 1
  assessment 18–19
  communication 32, 38
  discharging 6
  ID 4, 5, 10
  information management 8–10, 17
  management 2, 14
  see also dying patients; elderly patients;
        medical patients; surgical patients
patients' families
  communication 32–3, 37, 91, 95
  consent for post mortem 95
pay 199, 202
Pay As You Earn (PAYE) 209–10
payslip deductions 208
PCs *see* computers
peak expiratory flow rate (PEFR) 175–7
pelvic inflammatory disease (PID) 67
pelvis *228–9*
pemphigus 81
penicillins 105, 191
pensions 209
peptic ulcers 39, 40, 41, 47, 76, 115
perforated bladder 171
perforated bowel 171
perfusion 35
  abnormalities 49
pericardial disease 127
pericardial tamponade 35, 75, 82, 83
pericarditis 47, 55
period pain 67
perioperative hypertension 71
peripheral arterial thromboembolism 121
peripheral neuropathy 57
peripheral oedema 88
peritoneal tap (paracentesis) 169–71
peritoneoscopy 130
peritonism 39, 40, 52, 76
peritonitis 171
permanent health insurance 208
personal folders 8, 10
pethidine 114, 125, 126, 136, **138**, 173
phaeochromocytoma 128–9
phantom limb pain **138**
pharmacists 99, 100

phenobarbitone 47, 61
phenothiazines 77
   overdose 61
phenytoin 47, 61, 62, **108**
phlebitis 58, 62, 78
phosphate enemas 51, 124
phosphates 46
   intoxication 47
photophobia 69
phytomenadione 107
Picolax sachets 124, 181, 182
PID (pelvic inflammatory disease) 67
pink puffers 144–5
pityriasis alba 81
pityriasis rosea 82
plain films 180–1
platelet transfusions 86–7
pleural aspiration 171–3
pleural effusion 157
   chest drain insertion 158
   investigations 132
pleurisy 47
pleuritic chest pain **138**, 162
pleurodesis 158
PND (paroxysmal nocturnal dyspnoea) 73
pneumococcal septicaemia 191
pneumonia 47, 49, 58, 59, 76, 82
   aspiration 105
   atypical 113
   investigations 131–2
pneumothorax 35, 75, 82, 83, 84, 126
   chest drain insertion 157–8
   and chest pain 47, 48
   and liver biopsy 125
   and pleural aspiration 173
   tension 76, 156
poisons information 18, 215
polyarthritis, investigations 132
polycythaemia rubra vera 74
polystyrene sulphonate resin (Calcium
      Resonium) 79
porphyia 84
post mortems 94, 95, 96
posterior ischaemia 55
postoperative care 192–3
postoperative confusion 49
postoperative hypertension 71
postoperative ileus 50
postoperative pain relief, day surgery 196
potassium 50, 79–81
   hypokalaemia, elderly patients 111

imbalance 63
infusion 195
levels 35
supplements 80, 81, 111
povidone 166
PR interval 53, 54–5
prednisolone 107, 116
pregnancy 76, 114
   and abdominal pain 22
   and leave 202
   and radiology 114, 180
   tests 189
preoperative checklist **188–9**, 192
preoperative hypertension 71
prescriptions, writing 100
presentation software 24
presenting complaints 117, 118
priority setting 2
procedures 140–77
   diagrams for patient explanations 190,
      223–30
   patient preparation 121–7
prochlorperazine 77, 125, 126, 173
procurators fiscal 96–7
professionalism 28
progestagen 189
programs *see* software
prophylaxis 51, 62, 116
prostatectomy 191, *229*
protamine sulphate 106
proteinuria 68, 70
pseudomembranous colitis 51, 105
psoriasis 81, 82
psychiatric disorders 21
PubMed 25
pulmonary embolism 35, 82, 83, 84, 105
   and chest pain 47, 48
   electrocardiogram 56
   and hypotension 71, 72
   ventilation perfusion scans 184
pulmonary oedema 49, 75, 83, 173
pulse oximetry 49, 72, 78, 82, 88
pulsus paradoxus 83, 84, 173
pustular diseases 81
pyogenic granulomas 82

Q waves 56
QRS complexes 45, 52, 53, 55, 158–9

radial artery puncture 141, *142*
radiation exposure 178–9

radioactive implants
  checks
    before cremation 94, 97
    before MRI 184
radioisotope scanning 184
radiology 40, 59, 178–84
  arteriography 183
  computerized tomography 180, 183
  contrast studies 181–2
  doses **179**
  magnetic resonance imaging (MRI) 131,
    184
  patient preparation 178
  plain films 180–1
  and pregnancy 114, 180
  radioisotope scanning 184
  requests 4, 178
  ultrasound 129, 182–3
ranitidine 64, 116
rashes 74, 81–2, 87
RBBB (right bundle branch block) 55
referees 205
referral letters 14–15
Registrar of Births and Deaths 95, 96
rehydration 114
renal biopsy 126–7, *230*
renal colic 21, 22, 126, **138**
renal disease 47, 70, 127–8
renal failure 49, 64, 70, 76
  acute 78, 87
  investigations 131
  late 74
renal parenchymal disease 67
renal stones *230*
renal tract disease 67
representation 199
  junior doctors 213
representatives, drug companies 204
respiratory depression 49
respiratory disease, and arterial blood gas
    interpretation 144–5
respiratory failure 81
  investigations 132
  type 1 (pink puffers) 144–5
  type 2 (blue bloaters) 145
respiratory function tests 173–7
respiratory investigations 131–2
results, normal ranges 218–19
Resuscitation Council (UK) 35, 37
resuscitation status 37
retinal detachment 57

retinal haemorrhages 70
retroperitoneal bleeding 41
reviews 27
rheumatoid arthritis 58, 192
rheumatological investigations 132
rib collapse 48
right bundle branch block (RBBB) 55
right ventricular function (RVF), abnormal
    157
right ventricular hypertrophy (RVH) 55
ring binders 4, 8
rosacea 81
rotas 200–1
Royal College of Radiologists 178, 180, **181**,
    192
Royal College of Surgeons 196
RVF (right ventricular function) 157
RVH (right ventricular hypertrophy) 55

salbutamol 72, 75, 83
salicylates, poisoning 18, 19
saline 85, 101, 111, 154
saline diuresis 46
savings, tax-free 210–11
SBE (subacute bacterial endocarditis) 60
scabies 74, 81
sciatica **138**
seborrhoeic keratoses 81
sectioning, for treatment refusal 20, 217
sedation 124, 126
  confusion 49, 50
  insomnia 73
  night 107
sedatives 49, 57, 73–4
self-care 198–214
self-discharge 13, 15, 30
self-discharge notes 15
self-mutilation 17–18
senior registrars, communication 29–30
senna 51
sepsis 44, 52, 66, 82, 88, 166
  and central lines 154
  and hypotension 71
  moribund patients 75, 76
septicaemia 105, 115
serial forms **12**, 13
serum samples 18
shifts *see* rotas
shingles 40, 56, 70, 74, 81, 116
  and chest pain 48
shock 44

shortness of breath 82–4
SIADH (syndrome of inappropriate ADH) 84, 85
'sick cell' syndrome 85
sick leave 203
sick notes 15
sick patient checklist 84
sick sinus syndrome 43
sickle cell anaemia 114–15
sigmoidoscopy 52, 124
sinus arrest 45
sinus bradycardia 43
sinus tachycardia 44
sinusitis 69, 169
sisters 31
skin atrophy 115
skin lesions 74, 81–2, 113
skull X-rays 180, **181**
sleep 72–4, 213–14
small bowel enemas 182
social work rounds 5
sodium 84–5
    retention 115
    urinary 88
sodium picosulphate 124
sodium valproate **108**
software 23, 24–5, 26
'special' nursing 32
sphygmomanometers 148
spinal cord compression/lesions 50
spirometry 173–5
spironolactone 79
splenectomy 191
spreadsheets 24
squamous cell carcinomas 81, 82
SSRVs (structured small round viruses) 52
ST segment 53, 55
staff nurses 31
Stain Devils 200
stains 3, 199–200
staphylococcal infection 60, 82
Staphylococcus aureus 78
    methicillin resistance 204
stenting 121, 122
steroid therapy 115–16
    acute illness management 115–16
    perioperative prescribing 186
    withdrawal 116
steroid-dependent patients 195
steroids 60, 66, 72, 78, 107
    injections 165

side effects 115, 116
stethoscopes 3
sticky labels 8–10, 185
stool softeners 51
stool specimens 52
streptococcal skin infections 82
striae 115
stroke 49
    elderly patients 111
    head CT 183
structured small round viruses (SSRVs) 52
student nurses 31
study leave 203
subacute bacterial endocarditis (SBE) 60
sub-arachnoid haemorrhage 61, 69
    head CT 183
subclavian vein cannulation 151, 153
subcutaneous injections 162
subdural haematoma 49, 61, 69
suicidal thoughts 111
    HIV/AIDS patients 113
    patient assessment 21
superannuation 208, 209
suprahyperglycaemia 61
supraventricular tachycardia (SVT) 44, 45
surgical patients 185–97
    anaesthetics 191–2
    clerking 185–6
    clerking sheets 186, 197
    consent 189–91, 196
    day surgery 196
    diabetes mellitus 193–5
    expected side effects after surgery 191
    information-giving 190–1, 196
    jaundice 191, 193
    marking 192
    oro-facio-maxillary surgery 196–7
    perioperative prescribing 186–9
    postoperative care 192–3
    preoperative checklist **188–9**, 192
    steroid-dependent 195
    theatre lists 192
    thyroid surgery 195
surgical protocol clerking sheets 186, *187*, 196, 197
sutures 177
    removal **177**
SVT (supraventricular tachycardia) 44, 45
sympathomimetics 44
syncope 57, 58

syndrome of inappropriate ADH (SIADH) 84, 85
syphilis 82, 130
syringes 102–4, 140–1, 194–5

T cells 113
T waves 53, 55, 56, 158
tachyarrhythmias 44–5
tachycardia 45, 58
tachypnoea 76, 83, 111
tape decks 6
tax 209–11
    allowances 210
    tax deductible items 210
    untaxed income declaration 210
team nursing 31–2
technetium scanning 184
teeth, notation 196
telephone banking 211
telephone numbers 8, 9, 10
temazepam 73, 108, 125, 183, 186
temporal arteritis 57, 69, 70
tenoxicam 135
TENS (transcutaneous electrical nerve stimulation) 138
tension headaches 68, 69
tension pneumothorax 156
terfenadine 74
terminal care 90–4
    breaking bad news 90–1
    drug prescribing 88, 93, 99
    ongoing communication 91–3
    pain control 91, 93
    support organizations 93–4
    symptom control 93
tetany 47
thalassaemia 41
theatre lists 192
theophylline 44, 45
therapeutic drug levels 107, 108
thiamine 62
thiazide diuretics 48, 61, 84
thioridazine 50, 84
thorax 223
thrombocytopenia 86
thrombosis 58
thrush 105
thyroid disease 129
thyroid imbalance 111
thyroid surgery 46, 191, 195
thyroxine 61
TIA (transient ischaemic attack) 57

ticarcillin 79
ticlopidine 82
timetables 10
tinea corporis 82
tinea cruris 82
tinea pedis 81, 82
tinea versicolor 81
tobramycin 108
total parenteral nutrition (TPN) 47
transcutaneous electrical nerve stimulation (TENS) 138
transfusion reactions 87
transfusions 85–7
    see also blood transfusions
transient ischaemic attack (TIA) 57
treatment refusal 113–14, 190, 217
    overdose 20
triamcinolone 165
triamterene 79
tricyclic antidepressants 50, 69
    overdose 19, 61
triglycerides 127, 128
trimethoprim 105
TRIPS (database) 25
trolleys 16, 30
    arrest 35
tropicamide 4
TTA sheets 13
TTO sheets 4, 13–14
tuberculosis 115
    investigations 132
tumours 58, 67, 79, 146
    colonic 41
    secreting 85
typewriters 6–7

UK Medical Directory 200
ultrasound 129, 182–3
untaxed income declaration 210
upper gastrointestinal bleeds 63–5
upper gastrointestinal endoscopy 122, 124
    complications 124
upper gastrointestinal tract 225
    investigations 129
urea 61
urinary retention 49, 87–8, 191
urinary system 230
urinary tract infection (UTI) 49, 58, 67–8, 76
    antibiotic treatment 105
    investigations 131
urine 87–8, 145–6
urticaria 81–2

UTI (urinary tract infection) 49, 58, 67–8, 76, 105

vaginal bleeding 67
vaginal infection 116
vaginal itching 115
vaginal thrush 105, 191
vancomycin 105
  therapeutic drug levels **108**
varicella zoster 115
vasculitides 58, 82
vasodilators 57
Venflon 76, 103, 148–51, 153, 171, 172
ventilation 35
ventilation perfusion (VQ) scans 184
ventricular aneurysm 55
ventricular ectopics 42
ventricular extra-systoles 55
ventricular fibrillation 52
ventricular strain 55
ventricular tachycardia (VT) 44–5, 52, 53, 161
verapamil 50
vertebral collapse 48
vesiculobullous diseases 81
villous adenoma 79
virus detection software 25
vision, sudden loss of 57
vitamin D
  deficiency 47
  intoxication 46
vitamin K 106
vitamin supplements 109, 114
vitiligo 81
Voltarol (diclofenac sodium) 21
vomiting 52, 76–7, 79, 80, 81, 166
vomitus samples 18, 19, 65
VQ (ventilation perfusion) scans 184

VT (ventricular tachycardia) 44–5, 52, 53, 161

wandering atrial pacemakers 42
ward calls 38–9
ward rounds 4–6, 17
  postoperative care 192–3
ward sisters 31, 32
warfarin 78, 105–6
  arterial blood samples 141
warts 81
washouts 18, 19
weight loss 69
Wenckebach phenomenon 55
Wessex Institute for Health Research and Development 27
Which? 211
Wolff–Parkinson–White syndrome (WPW) 44
  PR interval 55
women
  alcohol limits 109
  bladder catheterization 146
word processing 24
Wordperfect 24
work environment 6–7
World Wide Web (WWW) 26
wounds, delayed healing 115
WPW (Wolff–Parkinson–White syndrome) 44, 55

xanthelasma 81
X-rays 4, 192
  concerns 178–9
  and pregnancy 114
  screening 125–6, 168
  skull 180, **181**
  see also chest X-rays

Notes

JUDITH
CRAWFORD